Recent Results in Cancer Research

Fortschritte der Krebsforschung

Progrès dans les recherches sur le cancer

9

Edited by

V. G. Allfrey, New York · M. Allgöwer, Chur · K. H. Bauer, Heidelberg · I. Berenblum, Rehovoth · F. Bergel, Jersey, C. I. · J. Bernard, Paris · W. Bernhard, Villejuif N. N. Blokhin, Moskva · H. E. Bock, Tübingen · P. Bucalossi, Milano · A. V. Chaklin, Moskva · M. Chorazy, Gliwice · G. J. Cunningham, London · W. Dameshek, Boston M. Dargent, Lyon · G. Della Porta, Milano · P. Denoix, Villejuif · R. Dulbecco, San Diego · H. Eagle, New York · R. Eker, Oslo · P. Grabar, Paris · H. Hamperl, Bonn R. J. C. Harris, London · E. Hecker, Heidelberg · R. Herbeuval, Nancy · J. Higginson, Lyon · W. C. Hueper, Bethesda · H. Isliker, Lausanne · D. A. Karnofsky, New York · J. Kieler, København · G. Klein, Stockholm · H. Koprowski, Philadelphia · L. G. Koss, New York · G. Martz, Zürich · G. Mathé, Paris · O. Mühlbock, Amsterdam · G. T. Pack, New York · V. R. Potter, Madison · A. B. Sabin, Cincinnati · L. Sachs, Rehovoth · E. A. Saxén, Helsinki · W. Szybalski, Madison H. Tagnon, Bruxelles · R. M. Taylor, Toronto · A. Tissières, Genève · E. Uehlinger, Zürich · R. W. Wissler, Chicago · T. Yoshida, Tokyo · L. A. Zilber, Moskva

Editor in chief

P. Rentchnick, Genève

Springer-Verlag New York Inc. 1967

Immunological Aspects of Viral Oncolysis

Jean Lindenmann · Paul A. Klein

With 25 Figures

Springer-Verlag New York Inc. 1967

Professor Jean Lindenmann, M.D., Institute for Medical Microbiology,
The University of Zurich/Switzerland

Paul A. Klein, Ph. D., Department of Microbiology, College of Medicine,
University of Florida, Gainesville, Florida/USA

Sponsored by the Swiss League against Cancer

ISBN-13: 978-3-642-87046-0   e-ISBN-13: 978-3-642-87044-6
DOI: 10.1007/978-3-642-87044-6

Table of Contents

Work supported in part by NIH General Research Support Grant FR-05062-03, Research Grant AI 1302-08 and Training Grant TI AI 128-04.

"...in pursuit of those far mysteries we dream of, or in tormented chase of that demon phantom that, some time or other, swims before all human hearts; while chasing such over this round globe, they either lead us on in barren mazes or midway leave us whelmed."

Herman Melville (1851)
"Moby Dick"

Introduction

The immunobiologist faces most perplexing problems when dealing with neoplastic tissue. At first sight it seems almost impossible that malignant cells with their grossly abnormal morphology and behavior should not be in some way antigenically different from normal cells. If they are antigenically different, why do they fail to evoke an immune response? Or if they do evoke an immune response, why do they continue to grow?

In the following pages we wish to draw the attention of the reader to a potentially useful model which approaches the problem in a novel way. We realize that the work to be reported is not cancer research in a classical sense and does not fit the general heading of this monograph series. However, in a subject like cancer research, which after countless high-flying and hopeful starts has lost itself so many times in "barren mazes" [1], we feel that any avenue which shows the field in a new perspective is worth taking note of.

Our system evolved from the chance observation that inbred A2G mice were naturally resistant to certain myxoviruses. When viral oncolysis of a transplantable tumor was performed in such mice using a tumor-adapted strain of influenza virus, many animals survived and were cured of the tumor. Such postoncolytic survivors proved to be highly immune to challenges with the same and other transplantable tumors.

Studies on the nature of this tumor immunity revealed that it was mediated by circulating antibodies. Protection experiments showed that not all strains of mice could be passively protected against tumor challenge. Use of another oncolytic agent, reovirus type 3, pointed out that long term survival was only seen in those mouse strains in which passive protection with postoncolytic serum was successful.

Antibodies did not appear to be directed against known histocompatibility antigens. One antigen-antibody reaction which occurred using postoncolytic sera could be visualized by gel-precipitation techniques. This became the first reported

---

[1] We are referring to the notorious propensity of white whales to turn into red herrings.

mouse tissue alloantigen detected by this procedure. An antigen of cross-reacting specificity was revealed in tissue extracts of many other animal species.

We next wanted to learn more about the antigen responsible for induction of postoncolytic immunity. Extracts from virus-infected tumors were immunogenic, and both active and inactive fractions of such extracts were obtained. The growth of the virus in the tumor cells was studied with the electron microscope, in the hope that this might shed some light on the manner in which viral infection transforms a poorly immunogenic tumor into a highly immunogenic one.

We consider none of the questions which our work has raised as definitely solved. In fact, we are still working on many of the aspects alluded to above. When we embarked on a study of postoncolytic immunity, we were supported in this endeavor by our lack of experience in the fields of transplantation and tumor immunology. For in the eyes of a proper tumor immunologist, our work was handicapped from the start by the necessity of using so-called nonspecific tumors. Cancer workers dislike these tumors for two main reasons. One is that some of these tumors date back to a time when much early enthusiasm and an enormous amount of work had to be written off as the rules governing tissue transplantation became known. The death knell of this early phase of cancer immunology was sounded in a widely quoted review by WOGLOM (1929), who warned that "cancer research is a discipline requiring some apprenticeship and ... not everyone with an inoculating needle and a dozen white mice can plunge in and emerge with a discovery".

The second reason is that nonspecific tumors seem to remain unaware of the discovery of the rules of transplantation and persist in growing indiscriminately across histocompatibility barriers. This stubbornness in refusal to abide by universal rules is indeed infuriating, and it is tempting to relegate these tumors to the realm of uninteresting laboratory artifacts.

One might still argue that even these disconcerting tumors deserve our attention if only because "they are there". A more rational argument is perhaps the following. Some tumors transgressing histocompatibility barriers can be found under "field" conditions. Thus, a lymphosarcoma of the Syrian hamster, which occurred spontaneously in a hamster colony, was homotransplantable from the start and could be transmitted from one animal to the other by cell transfer through cannibalism or insect bites (COOPER et al., 1964; BANFIELD et al., 1965). It is true that the hamster will be dismissed by some as being itself not much better than a laboratory artifact. But there is another example of a spontaneously homotransplantable tumor, the canine venereal sarcoma. This tumor was observed under field conditions in the U.S.A. and in Japan. Different isolates of this tumor showed great similarities in their chromosome complements, which were strikingly different from the normal karyotype of the dog. It appeared that the tumor was spread by natural homotransplantation during venereal contact (WEBER et al., 1965).

The best justification for studying nonspecific tumors is their usefulness as models. It must, however, be made very clear what kind of models we may expect from such tumors. Let us perhaps first consider what features are to be demanded of any model. A model, of course, is never identical with the real situation which it is intended to illuminate. One might think that the closer the model resembles the "real life" situation, the better it is. We wish to suggest that this idea is not always correct. For the best approximation to the real situation is that situation itself, and no model is needed at all. Rather, a model should present certain features of the real situation in a grotesquely exaggerated manner. It does not matter if at the same time some other features are blurred or lost, as long as it is acutely remembered what features of the model are relevant to the particular study under way.

One very legitimate question which our model is *not* intended to answer is the following: Are tumors antigenically different from the normal tissue in which they originated? We shall briefly review the arguments which suggest that such antigenic differences indeed exist, but we shall not make use of our own work to decide the issue either way.

We shall instead turn our attention to the next question: Granted some tumors are antigenically different from their host, why do such tumors nevertheless grow? We propose to approach this problem with the aid of an appropriate model. What we want to study is malignant growth in spite of antigenic differences between tumors and hosts. As stated above, a useful model should exhibit these features in a grotesquely exaggerated manner. Thus the model tumor should grow fast from very small inocula, without signs of being checked by host defense mechanisms, and it should do this in the face of gross antigenic differences between tumor and host. These are exactly the features which we find in some nonspecific tumors, and it is in this sense that we shall interpret some of our results.

We have arranged the material to be presented in the following order: In Chapter I we give a brief review of tumor immunology, in Chapter II of viral oncolysis and in Chapter III of inborn resistance to viruses in mice. Chapter IV contains a more detailed review of our own work on viral oncolysis and postoncolytic immunity, including some unpublished material. In Chapter V we attempt a general discussion of the subject in the light of our results.

I. Tumor Immunity. A Brief Review

The experiments which we shall describe at some length in chapter IV deal with the ability of mice to overcome, by immunological means, the implantation of otherwise lethal numbers of tumor cells. Such phenomena clearly belong to the realm of tumor immunology. The transplantation of tumors usually follows the same rules that govern the transplantation of normal tissues. Failure to realize this has lead to some confusion in the past. In the words of MEDAWAR: "Nearly everyone who supposed that he was using transplantation to study tumors was in fact using tumors to study transplantation — not always to very good effect." (MEDAWAR, 1958). We have already indicated in the introduction that we have more or less inadvertently stumbled into this complicated and controversial field. Fortunately for us, the subject abounds in excellent reviews. We shall attempt in the following pages to discuss some of the facets of transplantation immunology which we believe to be pertinent to our problems. We must, however, refer the reader to a number of review articles for a more balanced account: Transplantation immunity (AMOS, 1962; HELLSTRÖM and MÖLLER, 1965); Transplantation antigens (AMOS, 1964); Tumor-specific antigens (OLD and BOYSE, 1964; SJÖGREN, 1965); Immunocompetent cells

(Gowans and McGregor, 1965); Antibody and graft rejection (Stetson, 1963); Enhancement (Voisin, 1963; Kaliss, 1965); Tolerance (Dietrich, 1964 a); Carcinogenesis (Potter, 1964; Temin, 1966).

Tumor Immunity of the Allograft Type

Transplantation or allograft (formerly homograft) immunity deals with the acceptance or rejection of tissues grafted between individuals within one species. It is governed by the occurrence of antigenic determinants, called histocompatibility antigens, on the cells of the graft and on the cells of the host. Thus, a graft bearing histoincompatible antigens will be rejected by the recipient in a period of time generally reflecting the immunogenic strength of the antigen(s) by which donor and recipient differ. "Strong" antigenic differences will induce rapid rejection of the graft, whereas "weak" differences will result in rejection after a much longer time.

The antigens residing in or on cells are themselves governed by histocompatibility loci which are inherited according to genetic rules. The best studied loci belong to the mouse. It has been estimated that there are at least 15 loci in the mouse concerned with the synthesis of the cellular products we detect as histocompatibility or transplantation antigens. These loci direct the synthesis of such cellular components in both the normal and neoplastic tissues of all organs. Thus, tumors generally contain the same transplantation antigens as do their normal tissue counterparts. It was this finding that greatly simplified the genetic analysis of homograft immunity in the mouse (Snell, 1948).

Thirteen of the histocompatibility loci have been detected experimentally in the mouse (Amos, 1964; Snell, 1965). The best characterized of these loci is the H-2 which has 20 known alleles. These alleles direct the synthesis of over 30 antigenically distinct products. These products have variously and still tentatively been characterized as insoluble lipoproteins (Davies, 1962; Kandutsch and Stimpfling, 1963), or water soluble molecular species (Kahan, 1965; Haughton, 1965). H-2 antigens have been reported to reside primarily on the cell membrane (Mishell et al., 1963) or within the microsomal fraction of cells (Manson et al., 1963). Some are detected by procedures measuring the various reactions of specific mouse allo-antibody with the antigens.

The nature of the immunity which develops following the inoculation or grafting of histoincompatible normal tissue or tumor into an immunocompetent recipient has been a matter of much debate. Some investigators feel that homograft immunity is mediated by immunoglobulins in the serum (Stetson, 1963), while others insist that it is chiefly mediated by sensitized lymphocytes (Strober and Gowans, 1965). Most likely the contribution of cellular and humoral elements to the observed immunity varies with the system and with the time when the observation is made (Pérez-Tamayo and Kretschmer, 1965).

Indeed, the mechanisms of transplantation immunity may be more complex than we imagined. Thus, antibody to surface antigens can actually inhibit the cytotoxic action of lymphoid cells on target tissue (E. Möller, 1965 a). Also "normal", non-immune lymphoid cells seem to be capable of destroying histoincompatible targets (Hellström et al., 1965; Möller and Möller, 1965; Ginsburg and Sachs, 1965). Macrophages as well as lymphocytes seem capable of destroying target tissue in the presence of specific antibody (GRANGER and WEISER, 1966; BENNETT, 1965). Those who advocate the role of humoral substances must be aware of the presence of non-immunoglobulin moieties in serum which might complicate and obscure their interpretations of the observed immunity (BROOME, 1963).

The mechanism by which an antigen initiates an immune response in an immunologically competent system is puzzling (NOSSAL, 1965). Both the charge of the antigen (SELA and MOZES, 1966) and the incorporation of the antigen into an adjuvant seem to be significant factors influencing the immunogenicity of soluble antigens (FREUND, 1956; WHITE, 1963; DIETRICH, 1964 b). Particulate states of antigens are more highly immunogenic than non-particulate states (NOSSAL, 1965). An unknown mechanism permits the host's cells to recognize the foreign antigen (BOYDEN, 1962 a). This probably involves humoral factors which promote a chemotactic effect thereby attracting more host cells to the graft bed (BOYDEN, 1962 b). There is some evidence that intracellular degradation of antigen within phagocytic cells is essential for the initiation of the immune response (UHR and WEISSMANN, 1965; GILL and COLE, 1965). However, both macrophages and polymorphonuclear leucocytes may destroy much of the immunological reactivity of the antigen (COHN, 1963; PERKINS and MAKINODAN, 1965).

Macrophages are perhaps primarily concerned with degrading the antigens of the donor cell and complexing them with RNA (FISHMAN and ADLER, 1963; ASKONAS and RHODES, 1965). In some unknown way this RNA-antigen complex is able to "tell" antibody producing cells to make specific antibody complementary to the antigenic determinant. The informational ability seems to be strain specific among various inbred mouse strains (COHEN et al., 1965).

Not all histoincompatible grafts, however, are rejected by recipient hosts. Thus a fraction of *H-2* incompatible mouse erythrocytes injected into isoimmune hosts was capable of surviving (G. MÖLLER, 1965). This was attributed not to the presence of resistant cells in the original population but to a mechanism whereby the interaction of antibody and components of normal mouse serum somehow converted susceptible cells to resistance. The phenomenon of immunological enhancement has been well documented (KALISS, 1965). This seems to play an important role in supporting the growth of incompatible tumors (E. MÖLLER, 1965 b). The classical experiments on acquired immunological tolerance revealed yet another mechanism whereby incompatible cells might persist for long periods in their hosts (BILLINGHAM et al., 1953). The loss of antigenic characteristics enables some transplantable tumors to transgress otherwise insurmountable histocompatibility barriers (MÖLLER, 1964). Genetic characteristics of the host may prevent it from responding to the incompatible donor cells. Certain strains of mice, for example, show no antibody production against specific determinants of synthetic polypeptide antigens (McDEVITT and SELA, 1965; PINCHUCK and MAURER, 1965). Perhaps some hosts make antibody with such a low binding constant that the biologic activity of the molecule is greatly reduced (SISKIND and EISEN, 1965). Yet other hosts may contain target antigens in common with the donor tissue and thus cannot maintain effective circulating levels of specific antibody (AMOS, 1955). All of these provide mechanisms by which histoincompatible cells (normal or neoplastic) could escape the immune defenses of the host. Their possible role in explaining the persistence of histoincompatible tumor cells in afflicted hosts will be discussed later.

Tumor Immunity of the Tumor Specific Type

The preceding section provided evidence that:

a) Transplantation antigens are distinct physico-chemical entities present in or on both normal and malignant cells of all mouse strains;

b) transplantation antigens can induce in immunocompetent hosts transplantation immunity with both humoral and cellular characteristics;

c) there are known mechanisms by which a histoincompatible tumor can escape immune defenses in an allogeneic host.

We can now turn to the problem of immunity to tumors containing tumor-specific antigens.

New cellular components have been detected in tumors induced by chemicals and in tumors and leukemias induced by viruses (PREHN, 1965; OLD and BOYSE, 1965). Most of these "new antigens" have been detected in tumor-bearing rodents (hamsters, rats and mice) using either the *in vivo* "transplantation resistance" phenomenon or *in vitro* serological techniques. Several workers have also reported the existence of distinctive antigens in human neoplasms (MCKENNA et al., 1962; GOLD and FREEDMAN, 1965).

Tumors induced with chemicals such as methylcholanthrene and benzo [a] pyrene contain unique antigens which persist for many transplant generations (PREHN and MAIN, 1957; KLEIN et al., 1960). Similar antigens can be found in tumors induced by physical means, such as the implantation of cellophane films (KLEIN et al., 1963). Most workers have found that tumors induced by such chemical and physical procedures do not cross react with each other. However, there are scattered reports that this may not be true in all cases (PREHN, 1965).

The possiblity that virus-induced tumors might possess specific antigens was discussed by LURIA (1959). Polyoma virus (HABEL, 1961; SJÖGREN et al., 1961), various adenovirus types (TRENTIN and BRYAN, 1964), Simian virus 40 (KOCH and SABIN, 1963), and the Rous sarcoma virus in mice (JONSSON and SJÖGREN, 1966) are all capable of eliciting resistance in adult animals to transplantation of the corresponding virus-induced tumors.

Five different antigenic types have been found in the case of leukemias in the mouse (OLD and BOYSE, 1965). Among leukemias induced by well characterized viruses, two distinct antigenic classes can be recognized. The Gross (passage A) virus induces an antigen (G) which is distinct from the antigens induced by the Friend, Moloney, and Rauscher viruses (FMR antigen) (OLD et al., 1965). The mammary leukemia antigen (ML) is shared by certain leukemias and mammary tissues infected with the mammary tumor virus (STUCK et al., 1964 a). The E antigen is found in the EL4 tumor and in leukemias which develop in old C57BL mice. Finally, the thymus leukemia antigen (TL) can be found in many leukemias for which no etiologic agent has been identified. This antigen is our first example of a tumor-specific antigen with its origin in the normal genome of the host, and we shall return to it later (p. 7). The chemical and physical nature of the tumor-specific antigens of chemically induced and virus-induced tumors is at present unknown. Once induced they persist for many transplant generations in syngeneic hosts bearing such tumors. One report describes the presence of soluble antigens of virus induced leukemias in the serum of animals with primary or transplanted leukemias (STUCK et al., 1964 b). These soluble antigens had the same serological specificity as the cellular antigens found on leukemic cells. This observation allowed the serological distinction of "high-incidence" leukemic mouse strains long before leukemia manifested itself.

It is quite clear then that neoplastic cells often contain serologically distinct antigenic determinants apparently absent from corresponding normal tissue. We must now seek some explanation for the failure of the immune mechanisms of the host to reject these clearly histo-incompatible cell types.

One recent experiment provides direct evidence that the host *is* capable of mounting an immune response against its own primary tumor (MIKULSKA et al., 1966). The authors suggest that failure of the host to eliminate the tumor is due to the exhaustion of the host's supply of immune lymphocytes. This suggestion, if validated, would fit the known facts concerning the essential role of lymphocytes in the immune response (GOWANS et al., 1962; McGREGOR and GOWANS, 1963).

It may be that many hosts actually enhance the growth of their tumors by responding to them with antibody formation (KALISS, 1965). It has been suggested that the type of antibody produced during the immune response may critically affect the occurrence of the enhancement phenomenon (BLOCH, 1965).

Immunological tolerance may play a significant role in preventing hosts from responding to tumor cells (DIETRICH, 1964 a). However, it most probably does not explain the well known differences in the susceptibility of newborn and adult animals to oncogenesis by most viruses (OLD and BOYSE, 1965).

At least two systems provide examples of tumor specific antigens which in reality exist either permanently or transiently as antigenic components of normal cells. One of these is the TL (thymus-leukemia) antigenic system of the mouse (OLD and BOYSE, 1965). In strains possessing the antigen, it is found solely in the thymus. The TL antigen, however, appears sometimes in the leukemias of mice lacking the antigen in their thymuses. Thus, it is an organ-specific isoantigen which appears as a leukemia specific tumor antigen in the TL positive leukemias of TL negative mice. All mice seem to have the genetic information for the synthesis of the TL antigen, but not all mice express it. During leukemogenesis in TL negative mice synthesis of the antigen is derepressed. Most intriguing was the finding that TL positive leukemias were not inhibited in immunized TL negative mice containing high levels of cytotoxic TL antibody. Further investigation revealed that the TL antigen actually disappeared from TL positive leukemia cells growing in immunized hosts (OLD and BOYSE, 1965). It would reappear in such leukemia cells upon passage in nonimmunized hosts. This phenomenon, termed antigenic modulation, may be an important mechanism by which tumor cells can escape from the immune defenses of the host.

The finding that dormant genetic loci are activated following the oncogenic event is quite important. The production of hormonal substances by nonendocrine tumors (BOWER and GORDEN, 1965) and of embryonal α-globulin by mouse hepatomas (ABELEV et al., 1963) are further examples of activation of genetic loci. A similar phenomenon perhaps explains the ability of placental tissue to immunize against Yoshida sarcoma (LUND, 1960).

When the oncogenic agent activates loci determining the structure of potentially alloantigenic targets we may be faced with many difficult problems. Such newly activated antigenic determinants might for example upset the mechanism by which the host decides what is self and what is foreign (DAMESHEK, 1965; VAUGHN, 1965). The reverse situation, loss of antigen, has been variously reported (e. g. TEE et al., 1964). The loss of an antigenic component does not, however, necessarily reflect deactivation or deletion of the genetic locus controlling its synthesis. It could simply result from the additional synthesis of an adjacent or superimposable antigenic determinant masking the immunologically reactive portion of the first antigen.

GOLD and FREEDMAN (1965) reported an experiment which provides our second example of tumor specific antigens which are actually products of the normal genome of the host. They found that normally occurring tumors of the gastrointestinal system of man contained a tumor-specific antigen. This antigen was not detectable in the tumors of other systems or in normal tissues of any adult organ system. The antigen thus appeared to be a system-specific tumor antigen. However, they soon found that human embryonic and fetal gut, liver, and pancreas obtained during the first two-thirds of gestation contained the antigen. It could not be detected in organs obtained during the last third of the gestation period. They called the antigen a "carcinoembryonic" antigen. They reasoned that the oncogenic process in the gastro-intestinal system of man had reactivated the synthesis of cellular components which had been present during the early development of that system.

If such carcinoembryonic antigens are really potentially vulnerable targets of the immune response of the host, then why are they not "attacked" more frequently? One possibility is that the host is tolerant of them because of its *in utero* experience with these antigens. Perhaps this tolerance is maintained by the continued production of these antigens during "minor" oncogenic incidents. These incidents can be dealt with by auxiliary nonimmune defense mechanisms such as allogeneic inhibition (HELLSTRÖM et al., 1965). Should the auxiliary mechanisms break down then the full blown neoplastic disease is able to manifest itself. Alternatively we could imagine that an almost immediate immune response is mounted against these antigens, but that they are protected by an enhancement phenomenon.

Finally we must consider the possibility that these antigens are incidental by-products of the oncogenic process without offering vulnerable targets for immune attack. We know little about the role of histocompatibility antigens and tumor specific antigens in the economy of the cell. It is therefore difficult to ascribe a function to carcinoembryonic determinants in the economy of tumor cells. They are perhaps reactivated because of their functional role during embryonic development in the free movement of undifferentiated cells across one another. They would thus be surface components which are non-reactive in the phenomenon of contact inhibition and might be useful to cancer cells growing in an adult animal (ABERCOMBIE and AMBROSE, 1962; CARTER, 1965).

The ability of animals to make antibodies against a wide range of "self" components probably means that they may not in general lack the structural information for antibody production against carcinoembryonic antigens. NELSON (1965) has proposed a theory of transplantation immunity which requires, in fact, that antibodies always be synthesized against antigenic determinants of host cells. These host antigens would themselves cross-react with the target antigens of the graft. In an immune response, the antibodies bound to host targets would exchange places and bind to the graft targets for which they have a higher affinity. Although Nelson has some evidence that the anti-Forssman antibody can exchange in this manner, we have no knowledge of this phenomenon playing a role in tumor immunity. If it does, however, we might imagine a mechanism explaining the failure of many host's anti-tumor defenses. If the affinity of the antibody for the host cell antigen is greater than its affinity for the carcinoembryonic target, then the antibody will fail to exchange places. The host would thus have responded with specific antibody production but to no avail.

If some potential antigens of tumor cells are such that they are completely destroyed by intracellular digestion within polymorphonuclear leucocytes and macrophages they might fail to elicit cellular or humoral responses altogether. We may have to search for such antigens by finding ways to protect them from intracellular digestion while at the same time maintaining whatever immunogenic properties they have. This is perhaps an explanation for the antigenicity of alkylated tumor cells (APFFEL et al., 1966).

We have attempted in these few pages to cover a subject normally reserved for whole volumes. Our purpose has been to acquaint the unfamiliar reader with some of the complex problems in the field of tumor immunology. At the same time we have presented some speculative interpretations of recent findings. We hope that we have emphasized the needs of the tumor immunology field. Thus, it should be quite clear to the reader that much remains to be learned about the nature of cellular components with antigenic properties and their role in the economy of cells. Furthermore, we have presented some suggestive evidence that the dividing line between classical transplantation antigens and so called tumor specific antigens may be thin, indeed artificial when both are considered as products of the same genome. Viewed in this way, the study of cellular alloantigenic factors from whatever their source might contribute significantly to a better understanding of tumor immunity.

II. Viral Oncolysis: A Brief Review

The preference of viruses for specific cell types was recognized early in the course of virus research. It was relatively easy to conceive of certain viruses as being endowed with sufficient specificity to discriminate between normal and malignant cells. The idea was, indeed, tempting and not readily dismissable. If there should be any tool fine enough to distinguish between the normal and malignant state, a biological tool such as a virus, highly adapted to an intracellular environment, seemed to offer the best chances.

Ehrlich's chemotherapeutic concept of "magic bullets" capable of homing in on their targets would apply literally to a virus recognizing and selectively destroying malignant cells. The role of the virus would be that of a "super-scalpel" seeking out and eradicating individual cancer cells, however well hidden they may be. Failure of the virus to destroy all the cells would mean failure of viral oncolysis, just as failure of the surgeon to remove all cancerous tissue generally means failure of surgery as a cure.

Since the host usually reacts to the virus with the production of antibodies, the ability of the virus to effect complete oncolysis within the few days permitted for its development required rapid growth and fast spread by the virus. Accumulated experience showed that viruses which met these conditions were at the same time highly lethal for the host. The relatively few exceptions to this rule will be discussed below.

The vast amount of work devoted to viral oncolysis in the past 40 years has been extensively reviewed (MOORE, 1954, 1960; SIEGERT, 1955; SOUTHAM, 1960). The reader is referred to these excellent reviews for specific details. The experimental animal most commonly used has been the mouse, and the tumors were as a rule so-called "nonspecific" transplantable tumors which transgress the histocompatibility barriers of tissue transplantation. Since 1950, tumors were employed frequently in the ascitic form (KOPROWSKI, 1956). As for the viruses, there are probably very few that have not been tested for oncolysis at one time or another.

The Problem of Host Survival

We have already mentioned that the majority of successful oncolytic viruses were highly lethal for the host. The extent of oncolysis was assessed by morphological criteria (cytological and histological evidence of tumor destruction) and by a biological test in which the virus-infected tumor was transplanted into animals pre-immunized against the virus. Failure of the transplant to grow was taken as proof of its complete destruction. It was perhaps not always realized that even the second method might have failed to reveal the survival of a small fraction of tumor cells. For the bulk of the virus-destroyed tumor, what we shall call the "viral oncolysate", could conceivably immunize the fresh host against the tumor, so that the growth of small numbers of tumor cells having for some reason escaped destruction would be inhibited by an immune mechanism initiated in the new host. However, the eradication concept of oncolysis was so firmly established that a possible immunological reaction of the host was seen only in a negative aspect, as contributing to the early quenching of viral activity. A strategy was even outlined in which a battery of serologically unrelated viruses would be kept in store, so that injection of a second virus could finish the job of a first virus prematurely stopped in its evolution by antiviral antibody (SABIN, 1957). Nevertheless, it is not unlikely that early investigators were aware of a possible beneficial contribution on the part of the host. We shall exemplify this with LEVADITI's work on the oncolytic power of fowl plague virus. In 1931, HALLAUER had noted as a curiosity that fowl plague virus survived longer in tissue cultures from a mouse carcinoma than in similar cultures from normal mouse tissue. Six years later, LEVADITI and HABER described a necrotizing effect of mouse-virulent fowl plague virus on a transplantable mouse tumor. Tumor destruction was demonstrated histologically and by the failure of infected transplants to grow. Mice invariably died of the viral infection.

Evidently, the oncolytic effect of viruses would be more easy to evaluate and at the same time more dramatically demonstrated if long-term survival of the host could be achieved. LEVADITI and HABER, referring to the faculty of fowl plague virus to destroy tumor cells, wrote:

> "Pourrait-on utiliser cette faculté pour déclencher la résorption de tumeurs malignes, chez les animaux cancéreux, dans des conditions compatibles avec la survie de ces animaux?"

It is interesting that LEVADITI and HABER use the word "déclencher", *to trigger off*, tumor resorption. Perhaps this indicates that they did not expect the virus to accomplish all that was needed for the tumor to disappear, but that some sort of contribution on the part of the host was also required.

In view of the statement of LEVADITI and HABER as quoted above, one might have expected that the first examples of host survival after viral oncolysis would have been studied in great detail. This was the case only to a limited extent, however, and we can see the reason for this lack of enthusiasm. For in the meantime much had been learned about homograft rejection, and the fear of losing energy and time with irrelevancies loomed large. That this fear may have been justified is illustrated by the following examples.

SHARPLESS et al. (1950) tested a number of viruses against a transplantable lymphoid tumor of chickens. Some animals survived after virus treatment of their tumor and later proved refractory to re-implantation of the same tumor. This success was less impressive than might appear, since older animals rejected the tumor in a considerable proportion of cases spontaneously and were thereafter immune to re-implantation of the tumor. Hence the viral infection merely shifted an already labile tumor-host relationship slightly in favor of the host, thereby revealing the existence of a host defense mechanism probably of the homograft type. Nevertheless, this example is important in two respects. It shows the feasibility of some sort of viral treatment of tumors without lethal infection, and the potentialities of such treatment for the uncovering of host defense mechanisms.

Another example is offered by the work of GINDER and FRIEDEWALD (1951). Rabbit fibromas, induced by intracutaneous injections of Shope fibroma virus, could be destroyed by Semliki forest virus during the first 48 hours of tumor induction. The phenomenon was probably not due to viral interference, but rather to necrosis of tumor cells brought about by the superinfecting virus. Again, this is a system in which the host displays strong defense mechanisms which bring about regression of the tumors anyway.

Viruses suitable for oncolysis were obtained by one of three procedures:

1. Large numbers of virus strains from diverse origins were screened for oncolytic activity in several test tumors.

2. Viruses showing initially little or no oncolytic activity were adapted to tumors by serial passage.

3. "Passenger" viruses were isolated from transplanted tumors showing a sudden reduction in growth potential during their passage history.

If we try to evaluate the chances of these procedures to yield oncolytic viruses which would not be lethal for the host, the first seems to offer little prospect of success. For the observed oncolytic power of primary isolates probably reflects a state of adaptation to the host species rather than to the tumor. In spite of this handicap a few instances of host survival have been occasionally seen in large experimental series in which most animals died during oncolysis. This occurred unpredictably and the event was too rare to lend itself to experimental analysis. One report mentions successful oncolysis by Guaroa virus with survival of the mice, but all animals later succumbed to slowly growing subcutaneous tumors which apparently originated along the needle track of the primary tumor inoculation (KRULWICH et al., 1962).

The second procedure offers better chances. Starting with a virus which in itself need not be highly pathogenic for the host species, serial adaptation to the tumor might conceivably lead to a non-lethal, oncolytic virus. Such seems to have been the case with the successful adaptation of Newcastle disease virus to Ehrlich ascites tumor as reported by FLANAGAN et al. (1955). For instance, 14 out of 24 mice survived, although it is not stated for how long. No further details are given by these authors. This strain of virus was erroneously reported as lost (LINDENMANN, 1963). It has apparently been unearthed since, and survival of mice for 65 days after oncolysis has been observed (CASSEL and GARRETT, 1965). Neurotropic influenza virus has also been successfully adapted to growth in ascites tumors, but here death of the host is the rule (ACKERMANN and KURTZ, 1952; CASSEL, 1957). We shall consider this system in detail in the present monograph. It is interesting in this context that some viruses which do not usually kill adult mice upon intraperitoneal inoculation do so in the presence of an ascites tumor (CASSEL, 1957; FURUSAWA and CUTTING, 1960). The exact mechanism of this is not clear and may not be the same for all viruses.

The third procedure probably offers the best chances. If in the course of serial passages a transplantable tumor happens to be infected with virus of high mouse pathogenicity, the animal will be lost and it is unlikely that much effort will be devoted in trying to isolate the causative agent. If, on the other hand, a tumor picks up a virus which is neither pathogenic for the host nor measurably influences the growth of the tumor, such an event will not be readily detected, and in fact most, if not all, serially propagated mouse tumors do contain passenger viruses, about which very little is known. We are thus left with a third possibility, namely, that in the course of serial mouse passages a tumor suddenly changes its behavior, for instance by growing more slowly, by containing fewer cells per unit of fluid volume, or by exhibiting an increased percentage of inflammatory cells. If in such a situation a virus is isolated, this strain automatically is the result of a double selection for oncolytic activity coupled with negligible virulence for the host. Viruses which fall in this category are the oncolytic reovirus isolates of BENNETTE (1960) and NELSON and TARNOWSKY (1960). Disappointingly little experimental work has been published on this interesting system, which we shall consider in more detail later.

However, even such systems have their drawbacks, the most important one probably being that viruses which are accidentally picked up during tumor passages are likely to be latent contaminants of the colony of experimental animals being used. This brings additional complications, since some animals will be lifelong carriers of the virus, others will be highly immune, still others will be fully susceptible. It is therefore reasonable to look for other means of insuring host survival in the face of oncolysis produced by a highly pathogenic virus.

A straightforward idea which must have occurred to many investigators is immunization of the host against the virus. In all instances studied, this has proved detrimental to the spread of the virus, thus preventing oncolysis of an already established tumor and limiting infection of pre-mixed tumor-virus suspensions to those cells in which the virus had already penetrated by the time of introduction into the immune host. Little work seems to have been done with passive immunization, where the timing could be so arranged that oncolysis, at least in its initial stages, could proceed undisturbed. It is generally agreed that "serotherapy" of an established viral infection is unsuccessful, and this may explain the absence of pertinent reports.

Since many of the oncolytic viruses studied are neurotropic, local protection of the central nervous system might be sufficient to ensure survival. This has been attempted by the induction of interference with Newcastle disease virus in the brains of mice undergoing oncolysis by Bunyamwera virus (SPEIR and SOUTHAM, 1960). Here again most of the survivors seem to have developed solid tumors which eventually killed them. Protection of target organs with preformed or induced interferon during oncolysis has not been reported as yet.

The most promising approach so far has been the use of animals genetically resistant to the virus used for oncolysis. This has been done by A. E. MOORE with PRI mice supplied by A. B. SABIN. The tumor used was Sarcoma 180 and the virus was Russian spring-summer encephalitis, an Arbo B virus to which PRI mice are genetically resistant (see Chapter III). No detailed account of this work exists (MOORE, 1953; SABIN, 1954). At almost the same time, the group around Koprowski used a similar system, PRI mice and West Nile virus (KOPROWSKI and LOVE, 1953; KOPROWSKA and KOPROWSKI, 1953) and stated: "Infected mice surviving the 60-day observation period were found to be free from ascites and were apparently cured". In her excellent review from 1954, A. E. MOORE writes: "The ideal host is an animal such as the PRI mouse whose natural resistance allows viral multiplication and tumor destruction with no perceptible illness of the animal". Despite this relatively enthusiastic evaluation not much has been published since. The most enlightening report was again from Koprowski's group (KOPROWSKI et al., 1957), in which it was shown that PRI mice having survived oncolysis were highly resistant to challenge with several tumors, but the mechanism of this immunity was not studied.

III. Natural Resistance of Mice to Various Viruses

Before returning to the problem of host survival in viral oncolysis, it is necessary to present a brief review of genetically determined resistance to viral infections in mice. The phenomenon has been thoroughly studied in plants (HOLMES, 1965). Work on animals has been slow to start, perhaps because of the impression created by similar studies with bacterial infections, which showed that resistance was governed by a multiplicity of genes (GOWEN, 1960); present knowledge is summarized in a review by ALLISON (1965).

Arbo B

A colony of mice bred at the Rockefeller Institute was found to be resistant to yellow fever virus (SAWYER and LLOYD, 1931). This resistance was genetically determined, although the exact mode of inheritance could not be established (LYNCH and HUGHES, 1936). By systematic breeding, a line was derived which was resistant to St. Louis encephalitis and louping ill viruses; this line was designated VR (virus resistant) although it was by no means resistant to all viruses known at the time

(WEBSTER, 1937). In 1952 SABIN reported the very marked resistance of mice of Princeton Rockefeller Institute origin (PRI) to yellow fever virus (SABIN, 1952 a, b). PRI mice were also resistant to several other Arbo B viruses. The degree of resistance depended on the virus strain used and was, for instance, less pronounced towards the French neurotropic strain of yellow fever than towards the 17 D strain.

A simple mode of inheritance was found, resistance being dominant and governed by a single gene. Closer analysis revealed two factors contributing to the resistance. In PRI mice levels of virus replication were 10 000 to 100 000 times lower than in susceptible controls. This depression of viral multiplication was also evident in 5-day old baby mice. However, the young mice died, whereas adult mice survived. The operation of a cellular vulnerability factor was therefore postulated. This could be clearly demonstrated with challenge by French neurotropic yellow fever virus, which killed a proportion of adult PRI mice in spite of reduced levels of virus replication. Whereas the multiplication-depressing factor was inherited as a single dominant, the mode of inheritance of the cellular vulnerability factor could not be definitely established. PRI mice were resistant to several members of the Arbo B virus group, but fully susceptible to numerous other, unrelated viruses, including Arbo A. It was later shown that the genetic basis for resistance to Arbo B viruses was the same in Sabin's PRI mice and in descendents from Webster's VR line (GOODMAN and KOPROWSKI, 1962).

Resistance to Arbo B viruses was not determined by humoral factors, but was expressed at the cellular level. In brain tissue cultures from resistant animals the virus grew to a lower titer than in corresponding susceptible controls (WEBSTER and CLOW, 1936; WEBSTER and JOHNSON, 1941). An indirect approach to this problem confronts us with the first example of viral oncolysis in a genetically resistant mouse: PRI and "Swiss" mice received transplants of solid Sa-180 tumor. Six days later, Russian encephalitis virus (Arbo B) was injected into the tumor. Mice were sacrificed after 1, 4 and 7 days and whereas brain titers were 10 000 times higher in the "Swiss", the titers reached in the tumors were similar in susceptible "Swiss" and in resistant PRI mice. The conclusion drawn from these experiments was that resistance was a property of the cells and did not depend on some humoral factor (SABIN, 1954).

GOODMAN and KOPROWSKI (1962) showed that cultures of macrophages from resistant mice were less susceptible than similar cultures from susceptible mice. These workers also embarked on a breeding programme which aimed at the production of a strain of virus resistant mice congenic with one of the better known high-cancer incidence strains. The present status of this long-range project has been reported by GRÖSCHEL and KOPROWSKI (1965). The strain into which the gene for virus resistance was being systematically introduced by repeated backcrosses was C3H. Successive backcross generations were challenged with West Nile virus and the survivors (theoretically 50 % at each backcross) were mated with partners from the susceptible (C3H) parent strain. Eight successive backcross generations should theoretically yield mice differing from C3H by only a few genes, among them the gene for virus resistance. From Gröschel and Koprowski's report, it appears that this stage has not been reached yet, since within the supposedly congenic line sufficient heterogeneity remained to effect rejection of reciprocal skin grafts.

The existence of such congenic lines would open new possibilities for studying the mechanism of virus resistance. For only then would it be possible to make relevant comparisons between two strains. Let us suppose that an interesting difference exists between a resistant strain, such as PRI, and a susceptible one, such as C3H. For instance, let us assume one has more leucocytes than the other, or makes antibodies more rapidly, or forms less interferon. All these factors might be relevant to virus resistance, or they might be entirely fortuitous, like coat color. In congenic lines, such associations would have to be taken very seriously. Also, with congenic lines a number of experiments become feasible which are otherwise impracticable: Organ and cell transfers and parabiosis. At the moment, none of the experiments designed to clarify the mechanism of virus resistance is very convincing. Thus, THEIS et al. (1959) were able to increase the susceptibility of PRI mice to West Nile virus by injection of allogeneic spleen and bone marrow cells from susceptible donors. However, this was accompanied by a deep disturbance of lymphoid function as revealed by the occurrence of runting. VAINIO et al. (1961) compared interferon production in the brains of resistant and susceptible mice. They found that less interferon was produced in the brains of resistant animals. Since viral replication was also depressed in these brains, the low interferon titer did not necessarily preclude its contribution to the resistant state.

Mouse Hepatitis

A difference in susceptibility to mouse hepatitis virus between PRI and other mice was found by BANG and WARWICK (1960). Here PRI mice were highly susceptible. The genes for hepatitis susceptibility and Arbo B virus resistance segregated independently (GOODMAN and KOPROWSKI, 1962). It appeared that one or two genes governed susceptibility, and that resistance in this case was recessive. Cultures of macrophages from resistant mice failed to show the cytopathic effect characteristic of cells from susceptible strains. Susceptibility could be induced by adding extracts from susceptible macrophages to resistant cultures (KANTOCH et al., 1963). Cortisone also abolished resistance both in cultures and in intact animals (GALLILY et al., 1964). Thymectomy or the induction of a graft-versus-host reaction greatly increased susceptibility of resistant mice to MHV-1, a strain of low virulence, and macrophages from thymectomized mice were susceptible to the cytopathic effect of MHV-1 (quoted in ALLISON, 1965).

Ectromelia

Differences in susceptibility to mousepox among strains of mice had been noted by TRENTIN (1953). Contrary to the situation as outlined for Arbo B and mouse hepatitis virus infections, where resistance was exhibited at the cellular level, resistance to mouse pox seemed to be mediated by humoral factors. SCHELL (1960) suggested that C57BL mice, which were resistant to ectromelia infection, produced antibodies faster than susceptible strains. Macrophages from resistant and susceptible mice supported the growth of ectromelia virus equally well (ROBERTS, 1964).

Polyoma Virus

A similar situation perhaps holds for resistance of C57BL mice to polyoma virus. The pattern of inheritance is not clear. CHANG and HILDEMANN (1965) thought that susceptibility was dominant, whereas JAHKOLA (1965) favored resistance as an incompletely dominant character involving perhaps 2 genes. Early thymectomy abolished resistance (MALMGREN et al., 1964; MILLER, 1964). In vitro, C57BL cells were equally susceptible to transformation by polyoma virus (LAW, 1965). The somewhat earlier immune response exhibited by C57BL mice may be responsible for resistance not only to ectromelia, but also to polyoma virus, the Bittner agent and several leukemia viruses (JAHKOLA, 1965).

Leukemia Viruses

ODAKA and YAMAMOTO attributed differences in susceptibility to Friend leukemia virus to a simple genetic mechanism. Mice of the genotype SS were fully susceptible, mice carrying Ss had intermediary resistance, whereas mice with ss were fully resistant (ODAKA and YAMAMOTO, 1962, 1965). LILLY et al. (1964) noted that mice susceptible to leukemogenesis by Gross virus all had the histocompatibility factor H-2k. In crosses between susceptible and resistant mice of different H-2 genotype, offspring homozygous for H-2k had a much higher incidence of leukemia. Chromosome IX of the mouse contains in addition to the H-2 genes the gene responsible for an antigen present in thymuses and leukemias of certain strains of mice, the TL-antigen. LILLY et al. concluded: "... it is clear ... that this region of the genome is intimately involved in leukemogenesis in the mouse". TENNANT (1965) using a different system thought that "these results suggest that the H-2 constitution of the host may be a contributing factor to viral leukemogenesis, but is not the predominant factor".

Myxoviruses

Little was known about differences in susceptibility of mice to myxoviruses before 1962. Thus, LIU and BANG (1952) had reported that, depending on the mouse strain used, a variable proportion of animals developed encephalitis following intranasal inoculations of Newcastle disease virus. BRIODY et al. (1953) and BRIODY and CASSEL (1955) observed differences in adaptability of influenza virus to 3 strains of mice, and also differences in amount of lung consolidation, viral growth and frequency of death. KATO et al. (1961) found differences in susceptibility to the toxic action of intravenously injected influenza A virus. In spite of this, the general feeling was that mice responded rather uniformly to standardized inocula of mouse-adapted myxoviruses. This was particularly true of neurotropic variants of influenza virus (most of which were derived directly or through some genetic exchange from the first human influenza isolate, WS) and of fowl plague virus, an influenza virus of avian origin often virulent for mice upon primary isolation. Work with intracerebral inoculation offered the advantage that the infecting dose could be more exactly administered, so that failure of an animal to die could not be attributed to inadequate infection, such as might occur in intranasal inoculations.

In 1962 we reported that inbred A2G mice were highly resistant to the lethal action of neurotropic influenza A virus (LINDENMANN, 1962). The following picture has emerged from subsequent work (LINDENMANN et al., 1963; LINDENMANN, 1964; LINDENMANN and KLEIN, 1966; KLEIN and LINDENMANN, unpublished).

Genetics

Resistance in A2G mice was determined by a dominant gene, provisionally called *Mx*. The establishment of congenic lines was started by the systematic introduction of *Mx* into A/Jax and C57BL/6. No linkages have been found as yet between *Mx* and other known mouse loci, but this work is only at its beginning. The genetic constitution of strain A2G, which was quite nondescript when we started our work (*Committee on Standardized Genetic Nomenclature for Mice*, 1960) is now somewhat better defined: It is very probably *AA, bb, cc; H-2^a, Trf^b, Ig-1^e; Mx*. This genetic formula is interesting in view of the supposed origin of the strain A2G. In 1942, mice from Strong's strain A were introduced in England at Glaxo Laboratories. In 1950, H. Gruneberg inspected a few mice and thought that they differed sufficiently from A to require a new designation, A2G. It was suspected that at some time between 1942 and 1950 an "illegitimate" mating had occurred between an A mouse and a foreign mouse, probably an albino mouse, since an accidental mating with a colored mouse would not have escaped even a relaxed attention. A2G mice proved useful in the assay of pertussis vaccine (UNGAR and BASIL, 1957) and of certain hormones (STAATS, 1964). Strain A2G is currently being kept in various laboratories, such as the Laboratory Animals Centre (Carshalton, Surrey), the Centre de Sélection des Animaux de Laboratoire (Gif-sur-Yvette, France), the Antoni van Loewenhoekhuis (Amsterdam, Netherlands), Dublin Laboratories (Dublin, Virginia), and the laboratories of the present authors.

The genetic makeup of A2G mice reflects its mixed ancestry, several genes being common to A and A2G (major histocompatibility type, transferrin, immunoglobulin, coat colors) and others different (agouti, myxovirus-resistance, and probably minor histocompatibility loci). In addition, A mice show generally a high incidence of malignant tumors, whereas spontaneous tumors in A2G mice seem exceedingly rare.

The hypothetical illegitimate parent of A2G must therefore have been an albino mouse carrying the wild agouti allele and the gene for myxovirus resistance. Albino mice (homozygous carriers of the *c* allele) can probably only survive under laboratory or pet shop conditions. Hence it is likely that the illegitimate parent of A2G was a laboratory mouse, and it should be possible to trace occurrences of the gene *Mx* among other laboratory mice. Strangely, attempts to find *Mx* in other mouse strains have so far failed, although more than 20 strains were tested (LINDENMANN and KLEIN, 1966).

Mechanism

When resistance of A2G mice to neurotropic influenza virus was first observed, the possibility of a latent infection with an interfering virus was considered. This explanation was dismissed for the following reasons:

a) Conventionally reared mice and germ-free mice showed the same susceptibility to mouse-adapted influenza A virus; it would appear that the numerous microorganisms which contaminate conventional mouse colonies have little influence on the outcome of superimposed influenzal infection (TENNANT et al., 1965).

b) A2G mice kept in several countries and gnotobiotic A2G mice obtained from cesarean-section derived A2G mice reared by CFW gnotobiotic mice had the same degree of resistance as conventional A2G mice.

c) A Mendelian pattern of segregation was observed among F₂ and backcross offspring between A2G and susceptible mice.

All these observations were difficult to reconcile with the idea of an infective agent being responsible for resistance and favored a genetic interpretation.

Resistance was exhibited not only towards neurotropic influenza A virus, but towards many strains of influenza viruses of human and animal (swine, fowl) origin upon intracerebral or intranasal inoculation. It was independent of the process of mouse adaption often used to secure mouse-pathogenic variants of influenza virus (LINDENMANN and KLEIN, 1966). Among the myxoviruses, influenza A and B and parainfluenza 1 strains were shown to differ in virulence for A2G and other mice, but not Newcastle disease virus. Viruses not related to the myxovirus group were equally virulent for A2G and other mice.

Very little has been learned about the exact mechanism of resistance. In the brains of A2G mice neurotropic influenza virus multiplied, but reached a maximal titer hundredfold lower than in brains of susceptible mice. Qualitatively similar histological changes were produced in the brains of resistant and susceptible animals. Newborn A2G mice suffered lethal infection within the first 5 days of age; the period of susceptibility was prolonged in heterozygous F₁ mice. Resistance to lethal infection was not paralleled by resistance to the toxic action of large doses of influenza virus. No serum or brain extract inhibitors were found which could account for resistance, nor could resistance be passively transferred with serum. Preliminary results suggested that kidney tissue cultures from resistant mice were as susceptible to fowl plague virus as similar cultures from sensitive animals. Macrophages have not yet been tested satisfactorily.

Antibody levels developing after a dose of virus small enough not to be uniformly lethal for susceptible mice were lower in A2G than in control mice, probably a reflection of the lower viral multiplication.

An influenza virus strain adapted to grow in a transplantable mouse tumor reached high titers, whether the tumor was grown in resistant or susceptible mice. This experiment, inspired from A. E. Moore's work as reported by SABIN (1954), was the starting point for investigations reported in the next chapter.

IV. Tumor Immunity following Viral Oncolysis

1. The System

We have already mentioned that the most readily reproducible survival rates after viral oncolysis were obtained when use was made of mice genetically resistant to the oncolytic virus. What should now be done with mice which have survived oncolysis? Probably one of the most natural things to do would be to test such survivors for their susceptibility to re-implantation of the same tumor. Such challenge experiments were reported by KOPROWSKI et al. (1957). These workers found that PRI mice which had survived oncolysis of a nonspecific tumor by West Nile virus were highly resistant to challenge with the same tumor and several other transplantable tumors. The mechanism of this resistance was not studied, but the experiments gave rise to an interesting speculation known as the "cancer cure 1957". Since a very strong immunity to several tumors was induced by oncolysis of one transplantable tumor, it was thought that such an immunity could perhaps influence even a spontaneous tumor. Take a mouse with a spontaneous tumor. Inoculate it with a transplantable tumor. Induce viral oncolysis within this transplanted tumor with an appropriate oncolytic virus. The transplanted tumor will be destroyed and immunity to this tumor will develop. If now this immunity is also directed against the spontaneous tumor, the growth of the latter should be checked. Unfortunately, for this experiment to work, a spontaneous tumor should arise in a strain genetically resistant to the oncolytic virus to be used. The PRI strain was not suited to this type of experiment, because it failed to develop spontaneous tumors. It was for this reason that the development of a congenic, virus-resistant line of C3H mice was attempted. Successive backcross generations indeed showed increasing incidences of spontaneous mammary tumors approaching the level seen in C3H mice (GOODMAN and KO-PROWSKI, 1962), but the crucial experiment has not yet been reported.

The work of our group using a different mouse-virus system followed initially in the footsteps of Moore and of Koprowski. We felt that a thorough understanding of the type of immunity induced might be useful, and hence we shifted our attention from oncolysis proper to postoncolytic immunity. We wanted to express this immunity in quantitative terms using methods similar to those which have been standard practice for many decades in the study of immunity to classical infectious agents. It is surprising that this approach is not more frequently used, especially since individual mouse-tumor systems vary over such a wide range with respect to the "virulence" of the tumor, or, more precisely, to the number of tumor cells necessary to induce irreversible growth. Thus, in a recent publication, mention is made of an immunizing procedure which induced resistance to a challenge of 2.5×10^6 tumor cells, this being reportedly "several times the uniformly lethal dose" (APFFEL et al., 1966). Perhaps it might have been more useful to state that this was 10 or 10^6 LD_{50}'s. Since precise quantitation is more easily achieved with ascites tumors, we have used these tumors exclusively.

a) Growth of Nonspecific Tumors in A2G Mice

We have used three tumors in their ascitic form, obtained from different sources, and all three fell into the category of tumors highly virulent for A2G mice. We began our work with the Ehrlich ascites tumor, for the simple reason that the only tumor-adapted strain of influenza virus in existence had been adapted to this particular tumor (ACKERMANN and KURTZ, 1952). The Ehrlich ascites tumor, however, exists in at least two major variants and probably as many sub-variants as there are laboratories maintaining it by serial transfers.

The two major variants are known as the hyperdiploid Ehrlich-Lettré, and the hypotetraploid Ehrlich ascites tumor. The first has a characteristic chromosome complement described by BAYREUTHER (1952) with a total chromosome number around 45, two distinct marker chromosomes and a few minute chromosomes. When transferred under standard conditions with large numbers of tumor cells this chromosome pattern seems to remain remarkably stable. For instance, a strain of this tumor studied recently in China still contained the same two marker chromosomes and the minutes (Hsü LIAN-CHUNG et al., 1964). Another indication of the stability of the Ehrlich-Lettré karyogram is perhaps the following: In 1958, FELDMAN and SACHS described the chromosome pattern of an ascites tumor which they thought was a homotransplantable variant of the strain-specific tumor 6C3HED. This chromosome pattern was indistinguishable from Bayreuther's, and there are reasons to believe that this was not a coincidence, but that the tumor was actually Ehrlich-Lettré (HAUSCHKA, 1958).

In spite of this stability it proved possible to obtain several polyploid sublines from the Ehrlich-Lettré tumor (KAZIWARA, 1954). In general, the Ehrlich-Lettré tumors seem to be of low virulence, if one regards as a measure of virulence the number of tumor cells necessary to induce irreversible "takes" in 50 % of mice, as we propose to do. BOONE et al. (1965) compared a line of the tumor passed in tissue culture with a line serially transferred in mice and found in both cases an LD_{100} of approximately 10^6 cells. The polyploid variants isolated by Kaziwara (1954) were more virulent than the original tumor. These were obtained by a process intended to favor immunologic selection of tumor cells either intrinsically less immunogenic or less affected by the host's immune response. We might conclude from this that the Ehrlich-Lettré tumor maintains a constant karyotype by virtue of its relatively low virulence, which forces the experimenter to use large numbers of tumor cells at each transfer. The stability of the tumor might thus be guaranteed by a mechanism similar to that which stabilizes the virulence of BCG vaccine strains (GRUMBACH, 1956).

When in an ascites tumor the typical karyogram of the Ehrlich-Lettré tumor is found, it is probably safe to assume that this tumor is in fact a strain of Ehrlich-Lettré. Unfortunately, the reverse is not true. It is not certain that the various ascites tumors labeled "Ehrlich" and with chromosome complements in the hypo-tetraploid range are originally derived from Ehrlich-Lettré, or, for that matter, from any of the several tumors Paul Ehrlich had serially passed. Nor is it certain that all of them share at least a common origin. There is a gnawing suspicion that some of them might be closely related to the Krebs-2 tumor (HAUSCHKA, pers. comm.). Others may be offshoots of one of the Ehrlich-Lettré sublines. The origin of the Ehrlich strain we used for our first experiments illustrates the difficulties in tracing back such tumors: We obtained the tumor through the courtesy of Prof. J. Edwards. A thorough study of the replication of this tumor had been done some time before, and a chromosome number around 50 had been found (EDWARDS et al., 1960). This would place the tumor in the hyperdiploid category and perhaps close to the Ehrlich-Lettré. Unfortunately, marker chromosomes were not recorded. When after some time we studied the chromosomes of this tumor, they were definitely in the hypo-tetraploid range. Marker chromosomes resembling those described by Bayreuther were present, but similar chromosomes were also reported in certain sublines of the Krebs-2 tumor (HAUSCHKA and LEVAN, 1958). It is therefore impossible to decide whether the tumor is a hypotetraploid substrain of Ehrlich-Lettré, or a substrain of hypotetraploid Ehrlich which temporarily showed a reduced chromosome count. It is for the same reason impossible to categorically deny the possibility that this tumor has some affiliations with the Krebs-2 tumor which we have also used.

Not only do nonspecific tumors differ enormously between each other, but it is also almost certain that a single tumor behaves differently in different inbred strains of mice. Also, some tumors grow much better in one sex than in the other. It is therefore extremely important that quantitative indications be made on the virulence of the tumor (as defined above) for the particular mouse strain and sex used. The realization that some of these tumors are so virulent that occasionally the injection of a single tumor cell or of a very few cells into an adult host leads to progressive tumor growth would also help avoid some of the pitfalls awaiting the unprepared. For instance, supernatants from high speed centrifugation of such tumors have variously been claimed to induce tumors, the interpretation being that a virus present in such supernatants was the inducing agent. However, such supernatants do contain a few tumor cells capable of growing into tumors (MOLOMUT et al., 1964). Similarly, it is not unusual to find surviving cells in repeatedly frozen-thawed and mechanically disrupted tumors.

The two other tumors we have used, Sarcoma 180 and Krebs 2, both in their ascitic form, are less problematic. We have already mentioned a possible relationship between Krebs 2 and Ehrlich. Sarcoma 180 has, to our knowledge, never been suspected of identity with either Ehrlich or Krebs. Given the high virulence of these tumors, it is of course always possible to have laboratory pick-ups in the course of serial passage. We have therefore kept early passages of all three tumors in the frozen state. The antigenic similarities which interested us were already apparent in these tumors at the time they were received from reputable laboratories. We feel safe, therefore, in asserting that these antigenic similarities were characteristic of these tumors and were not the consequence of technical mishaps or clerical mistakes in our laboratories.

Table 1 shows a comparative titration of the three tumors in inbred A2G mice. All three LD_{50}'s are below 100 cells/mouse.

Table 1. *Titrations of Ehrlich, Krebs-2 and Sarcoma 180 Ascites Tumors in* A2G *Mice*

No. of cells inoculated [a]	EA	K-2	Sa 180
10^6	10/10 [b]	8/8	5/5
10^5	10/10	8/8	12/12
10^4	7/7	8/8	12/12
10^3	11/11	8/8	8/8
10^2	10/10	7/8	10/14
10^1	6/10	6/8	3/13
10^0	1/12	2/8	0/14

[a] Tumor cells were washed, counted in a hemocytometer chamber, appropriately diluted and inoculated intraperitoneally into adult female A2G mice.

[b] No. of mice dying of ascites / No. of mice in each group.

The growth of the Ehrlich ascites (EA) tumor was studied most closely. Routine transfers were done at weekly intervals in male mice with 10^6 twice-washed tumor cells. Washing was done with approximately 50 volumes of buffered saline and low speed (500 rpm) centrifugation. At several passage levels aliquots of tumor ascites were frozen in 10 % glycerol and kept at —70° C. A continuous line of the tumor was passaged in A2G mice to see whether a progressive change would occur. This line has now reached its 130th passage, and some changes in the behavior of the tumor do seem to have taken place (see below), although its virulence has remained the same. For titrations of virulence or for graded challenges the tumor cells were diluted in ten-fold steps from a starting dilution containing 10^6 cells/ml. The cell concentration of the starting dilution was established by hemocytometer counts. As an additional check for preventing gross errors in calculating the dilutions, we soon learned to recognize approximate cell concentrations by the turbidity of a suspension. For instance, cell suspensions containing 10^5 cells/ml were just barely turbid to the naked eye.

A quantitative estimation of tumor growth was attempted by counting the total number of cells in the peritoneal cavities at daily intervals. This method depended on our ability to wash out all or most tumor cells present, and was liable to error, particularly beyond the 5th or 6th day when invasion of abdominal organs began. Within the limits of this method, the tumor was found to grow exponentially with a doubling time of 14 hours up to the 5th day (LINDENMANN, 1963). Tumor growth was similar in random-bred ICR and inbred A2G mice. Histologically, the first evidence of organ invasion was obtained irregularly on the fourth, but always by the sixth day. The organs investigated were: Gut, abdominal wall, mesenteric lymph node, pancreas and spleen. The most regularly invaded organ was the pancreas.

In the organs which the tumor invaded there was no evidence of a cellular reaction on the part of the host (see Fig. 2). Smears made from peritoneal exudates revealed relatively large numbers of host cells, predominantly polymorphonuclear cells, during the first 24 hours after tumor inoculation. Whereas the tumor cells thereafter increased in numbers, the host cells decreased or remained stationary, being replaced by macrophages. From the sixth day on fewer than $10\,\%$ of cells were classified as host cells from their morphologic appearance on Giemsa-stained smears. From the first day of growth onward, less than $1\,\%$ of the tumor cells could be seen to have host cells attached to their surfaces (see section e, p. 45).

In some cases the tumor ascites became very bloody around the 6th to 8th day, and sometimes later. Death among A2G mice receiving an inoculum of 10^6 cells occurred between the 8th and the 20th day, and the distribution of deaths was not bimodal. Relatively few mice were inoculated with tumor and left to die during any single experiment, so that we do not have available large numbers suitable for statistical analysis. However, we certainly could not distinguish between a group of mice dying early with bloody ascites and another group dying late without hemorrhage, as reported by HARTVEIT (1961) — (see also SEYDAL, 1965).

When mice were inoculated with smaller cell doses, death occurred later. Thus, with an inoculum of 1000 cells, no mouse died before the 15th day, and some survived for 28 days. With inocula of 100 cells or below, some mice survived without ever showing ascites. When such mice were challenged 4 weeks later with 1000 tumor cells, they died in the usual time interval. We suppose that in these mice the first inoculum failed to grow. We have not observed the development of ascites with later regression in any untreated "normal" tumor bearing animals during the past several years.

A simple expedient for estimating the growth of the tumor was indicated by LETTRÉ (1941). It consisted of daily weighings of tumor-bearing animals. Since in the later stages a sizable proportion of the total body weight of a mouse was made up of tumor and ascitic fluid, the curves relating total weight to time gave a good indication of tumor growth. Such curves proved particularly useful for measuring the effect of viral oncolysis on tumor development (LINDENMANN, 1963).

We have devoted less time to the study of the growth of Sarcoma 180 and Krebs 2 tumors. Both seemed to behave in a very similar fashion to EA, with one exception noted below (p. 29).

b) The Oncolytic Virus

The virus which we have been using most extensively to induce oncolysis is a tumor-adapted strain of neurotropic influenza A virus developed by ACKERMANN and KURTZ (1952). Neurotropic influenza viruses hold a very peculiar position among influenza virus strains. The first was obtained by Stuart-Harris in 1939 from strain WS, the oldest human influenza isolate (STUART-HARRIS, 1939) and is known as NWS. From the same starting material, Francis and Moore succeeded in producing another neurotropic variant, usually called WSNF (FRANCIS and MOORE, 1940). Whereas non-neurotropic influenza viruses fail to multiply in mouse ascites tumors, NWS and WSNF do so to a limited extent (WAGNER, 1954). They also grow in a variety of tissue cultures which do not support growth of non-neurotropic influenza viruses (TYRRELL, 1955), and produce plaques in some systems (SIMPSON and HIRST, 1961). It has been suggested that these strains should be more properly called pantropic (WAGNER, 1955). They have a deficiency in their receptor-destroying equipment which prevents their ready elution from red cells to which they have attached, and their hemagglutinin is thermolabile and cannot be transformed to the indicator state.

Ackermann and Kurtz's virus was derived from strain WSNF. It had been passed 3 times in ascites tumor cells, one time in mouse brain, 51 times again in ascites cells and finally one time in the allantoic cavity before we received it. It grew well in our EA tumor, in the allantoic cavity of embryonated hens' eggs, and in the brains of ICR mice. It was not lethal for A2G mice even upon intracerebral inoculation of undiluted infected allantoic fluid. This of course was the prime requirement for its use as an oncolytic agent in A2G mice. We have called this strain WSA, the "A" standing for Ackermann. Infectivity titrations were performed in 10 day eggs (3 days' incubation at 35°C.) or by intracerebral inoculation of ICR mice. Hemagglutinin titers were measured by observing the sedimentation pattern of fowl erythrocytes in plastic trays.

In addition, we have done some experiments with another influenza A virus, fowl plague. We have passed the Langham strain of fowl plague (PEREIRA et al., 1965) ten times serially in EA tumors. Oncolytic effects resembling those observed after inoculation of WSA were seen from the 4th passage on. This strain, like WSA, is neuropathogenic for ICR mice and fails to kill A2G mice (LINDENMANN and KLEIN, 1966). The changes it produces in tumor-bearing mice are so similar to those induced by WSA that we shall not discuss oncolysis by fowl plague virus at any length. The interest of this strain lies in the fact that antiserum to WSA will not neutralize fowl plague virus and vice versa, and that fowl plague virus can be adapted to produce cytopathic effects in many different cell types.

Finally, we have done a number of experiments with an entirely different virus obtained through the courtesy of Dr. G. Bennette. This virus was isolated from an Ehrlich ascites tumor during passage of the tumor in Dr. Bennette's laboratory (BENNETTE, 1960). It has been characterized as a reovirus type 3 and produces oncolytic effects resembling those produced by WSA, but is without apparent pathogenicity for a number of strains of mice. We are grateful to Dr. L. Rosen for confirming the identity of this virus. The reovirus thus presents iteself as an interesting tool for studying postoncolytic immunity in many different inbred strains of mice inoculated with the same nonspecific tumor. We shall consider this system more fully in section g (p. 55).

c) Growth of WSA in EA Tumor and Oncolysis

Our usual procedure was to inoculate the oncolytic virus intraperitoneally into mice bearing 6-day-old ascites tumors, the tumors having been induced with 10^6 washed EA cells. This has proved to be a convenient schedule. When viral inoculation was performed much earlier, the clinical symptoms of oncolysis were less conspicuous, and a higher proportion of mice died later of slowly growing subcutaneous tumors developing at the site of the original tumor inoculation. When inoculation of the WSA virus was delayed beyond the 7th day, the disease accompanying oncolysis was of such severity that most animals died during its acute phase.

The dosage of the virus was also critical. An intermediate dose between 10^2 and 10^4 egg infective doses gave the most consistent results. Very large doses resulted in increased proportions of subcutaneous tumors, whereas with very small doses some animals escaped oncolysis altogether. Similar findings were reported by KOPROWSKI et al. (1957) with West Nile virus in PRI mice.

The growth of WSA virus could be followed by hemagglutinin and infectivity titrations. Fig. 1 gives the results of a recent experiment (HURWITZ and LINDENMANN, in preparation). The clinical symptoms of oncolysis were quite dramatic. A good objective measure of oncolysis was a rapid loss of weight (LINDENMANN, 1963; see

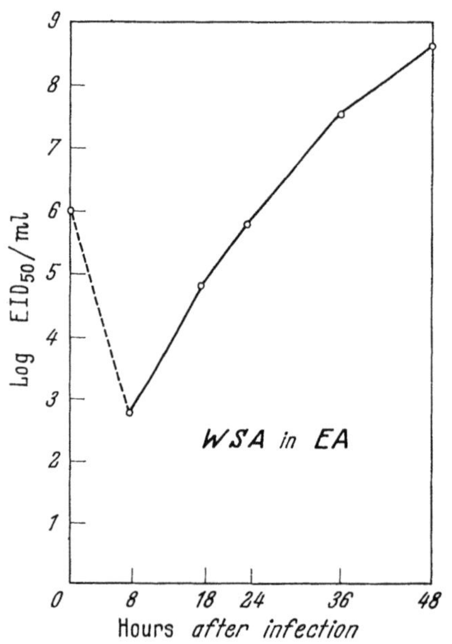

Fig. 1. Growth of WSA virus in Ehrlich ascites tumor cells. A2G mice were inoculated with 10^6 Ehrlich ascites tumor cells. Eight days later, WSA virus was injected into the tumor. Mice were sacrificed at intervals and the virus content of the ascitic fluid was measured by titration in 10-day eggs. Zero hour value was calculated from an estimated dilution factor. Haemagglutinin was not detected until 24 hours after infection, when it had a titer of 1 : 20. At 36 hours, the HA titer was 1 : 320, and at 48 hours, 1 : 800

also Fig. 18). The early stages of oncolysis were similar in ICR mice, which invariably died during oncolysis, and in A2G mice, of which a high proportion survived. The animals were obviously very sick, and remained with ruffled fur in a hunched position in a corner of the cage. The abdomen, which in untreated controls was distended with tumor ascites, caved in on the 2nd or 3rd day of oncolysis. When mice were sacrificed at this stage and their abdomens were opened, the tumor was no longer fluid but had solidified into large gelatinous masses. At later stages, all that remained of the tumor was a creamy layer on liver and spleen and whitish specks on intra-abdominal fat pads. During oncolysis a serious disturbance of peristalsis seemed to occur, the gut being vastly distended with gas and the anal opening smeared with liquid yellow feces. Some A2G mice which recovered from the acute phase of oncolysis accumulated during the following days black fecal masses in the terminal portions of the rectum and usually died. Mice which recovered from oncolysis and which were sacrificed 2 weeks or more after virus inoculation showed a normal peritoneal cavity. The gross appearance of oncolysis as reported above matches the description given by Nelson of reovirus-induced changes in an ascites tumor: "Mice ... often showed a white cellular membrane which partially covered the liver. Extension of the membrane into the mesenteric folds was accompanied by intestinal dilatation with rectal soilage or plugging. Chalky white areas of necrosis were also present in renal and genital fat deposits." (NELSON, 1964).

We have also observed similar gross changes after oncolysis induced by fowl plague virus. It therefore appears that these changes are not specific effects of the oncolytic agent used but reflect a sudden and massive destruction of tumor cells. The solidification of the tumor is probably due to coagulation of fibrinogen into fibrin. In electron micrographs of such solidified tumors we were able to identify strands of fibrin. This rapid coagulation is perhaps surprising in view of the fact that tumor ascites is very slow in coagulating spontaneously.

At the level of the light microscope, the changes brought about by oncolysis were no less striking. In smears of peritoneal exudates, nuclear disorganisation of tumor cells was clearly visible by 24 hours after virus infection. In smears stained with acridine orange and viewed in the fluorescence microscope, the yellow-green fluorescence of nuclear DNA was replaced in many cells by areas of red fluorescence. Smears from bloody exudates contained cells showing the phenomenon of hemadsorption, single tumor cells being surrounded by rosettes of erythrocytes. It was difficult to obtain satisfactory smears from exudates later than 48 hours after infection, probably because cells showing the most advanced stages of oncolysis were trapped within the solidified tumor masses.

Histological examination was most profitably done on sections of pancreas. Since the pancreas was regularly invaded by the sixth day when most oncolysis experiments were initiated, the invading portions of the tumor could be studied histologically. During the two days following oncolysis, additional tumor masses accumulated at the periphery of the pancreas and so became amenable to histologic sectioning. The overall picture revealed rapid necrosis of tumor cells without corresponding changes in pancreatic cells. This was not only true of A2G mice but also of virus-susceptible ICR mice. In fact, we do not yet know why the ICR mice succumbed so rapidly during oncolysis (LINDENMANN, 1963). In A2G mice, tumor cells underwent margination of chromatin, nuclear pyknosis, then transformation of the nucleus into a homogenous eosinophilic mass; finally, the whole cell appeared as a pale eosinophilic ghost. The entire process took less than 4 days. From the second day on, fibroblasts could be seen invading the necrotic tumor areas.

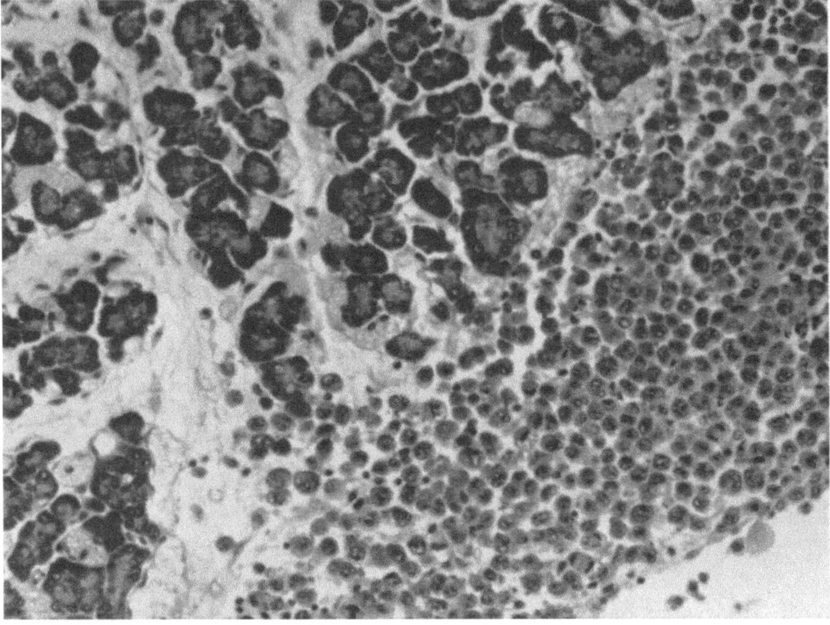

Fig. 2. Ehrlich ascites tumor invading the pancreas of an A2G mouse. Sixth day after inoculation of 10^6 tumor cells. HE stain, 250×

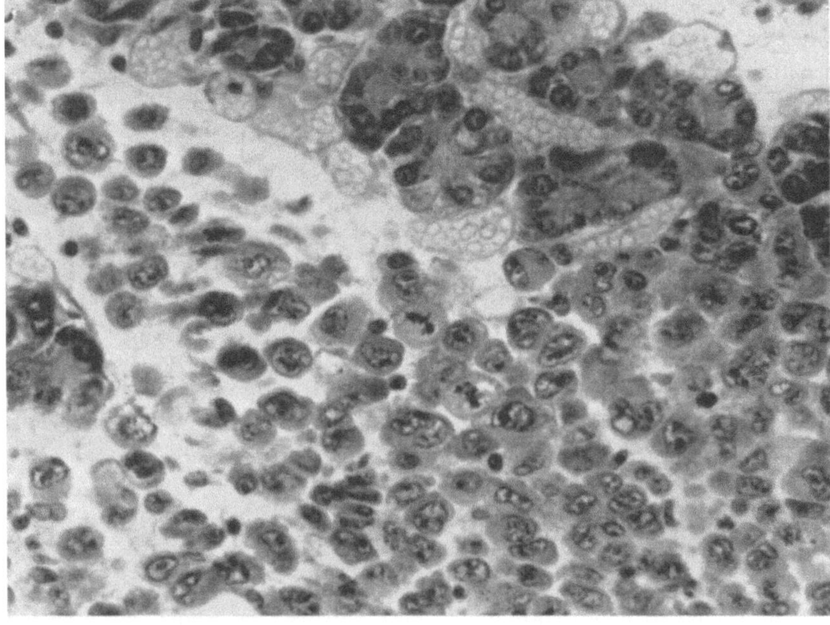

Fig. 3. Same as Fig. 2. 600×

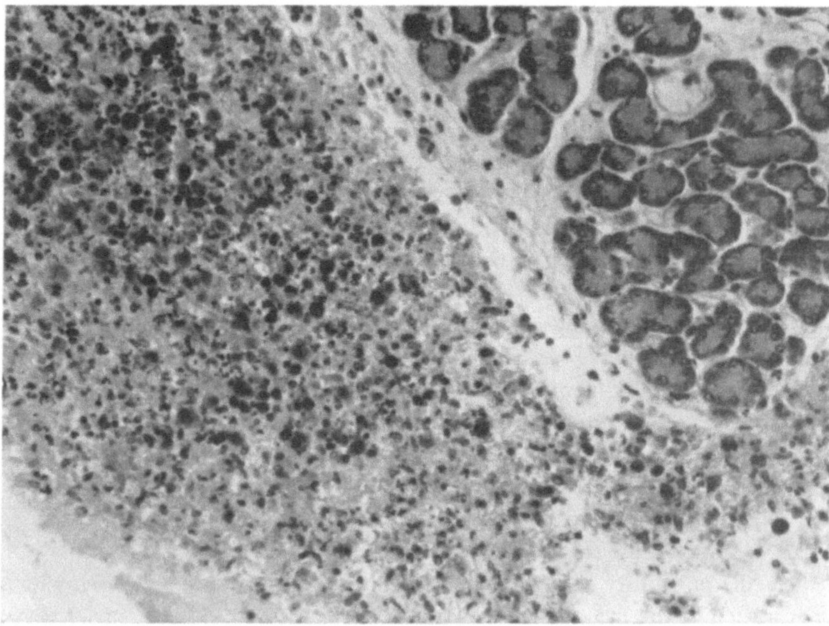

Fig. 4. Oncolysis of Ehrlich ascites tumor by WSA virus. The tumor was infected on the 6th day with 10^4 EID_{50} of WSA influenza virus. The mouse (A2G) was sacrificed 36 hours later and the pancreas was fixed for histological examination. Nuclear disorganization of the tumor cells without similar changes in the pancreatic cells is clearly visible. HE stain, 250×

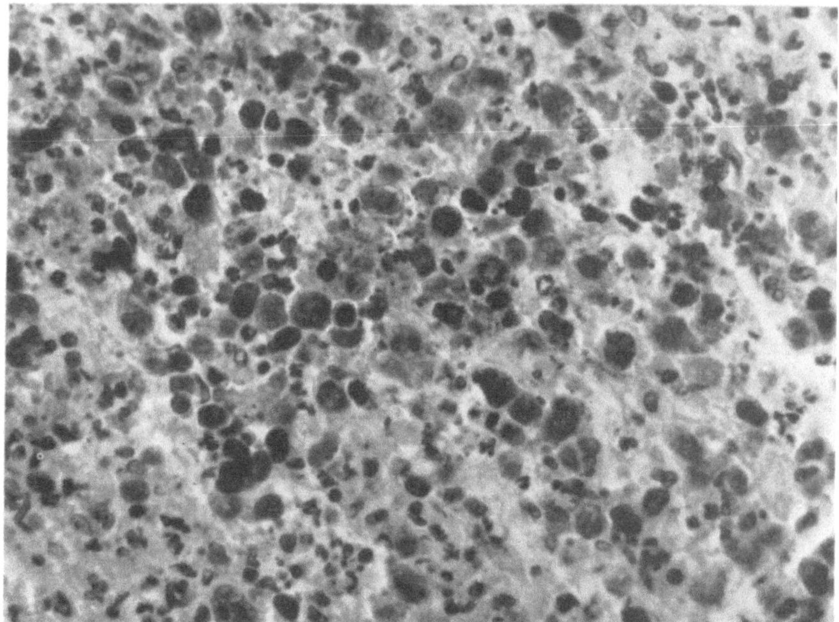

Fig. 5. Same as Fig. 4. 600×

From the inspection of many slides, it was clear that the process of tumor destruction started on the peritoneal side of the tumor. Thus, in early stages it was possible to see central islands of intact tumor cells within the pancreas surrounded by necrotic tumor masses. This was exactly the opposite of what was sometimes observed in 8 to 10-day old uninfected control tumors, where the center of a large invading tumor mass might be necrotic, probably because of insufficient nutrition.

Figures 2—5 give an idea of the changes associated with viral oncolysis.

At the level of electron microscopy, we were mainly concerned with the late stages of viral development, i. e. the process of budding from the cell surface. Study of the early stages of viral infection was rendered more difficult by the variously reported existence of passenger viruses in transplanted tumors which look very much like myxoviruses. We have seen only very few suspicious-looking particles in control uninfected tumors and many particles in tumors infected with large multiplicities of virus as early as 10 minutes after infection. However, we wish to reserve final judgment until we have done more work on these early phases (HURWITZ and LINDENMANN, unpublished). It is very difficult to be sure that one looks at control preparations with the same sustained attention one lavishes on infected cells, and we shall have to repeat this study with a "blind" safeguard against bias. Also, there is always the possibility that superinfection of a cell carrying a virus might trigger off maturation of the passenger.

All these difficulties could be ignored during the later stages of virus maturation, because the budding of particles at the cell membrane was so massive and obvious and had been previously so well illustrated for influenza virus growing in different host cells that a confusion with something else seemed most unlikely. Briefly, the particles of WSA matured at the cell membrane of EA cells much in the same manner as fowl plague virus or influenza virus does at the surface of allantoic cells (HOTZ and SCHÄFER, 1955; MORGAN et al., 1956). The virus budded as regular short rods with few longer filaments. Some cells seemed to produce enormous amounts of virus. Hemadsorption was of the cyto-hemadsorption type and no virus particles were found between adsorbed red cells and the EA cell surface (HOTCHIN et al., 1958). On negatively stained preparations, the virus had all the characteristics described for influenza A. Figs. 6 and 7 give an idea of the budding process at the surface of EA cells.

A strange and rather unpredictable event was the occurrence of subcutaneous tumors after the ascites had vanished. These tumors always developed at the site of the first tumor inoculation and probably originated from cells seeded along the needle track. It looked as if such cells were somehow protected against the virus. That the virus did not spread readily throughout the body was evidenced by the fact that ascites tumor growth was not affected by subcutanously injected WSA virus. In some cases such late subcutaneous tumors grew to the size of a pea and later regressed, or they grew progressively to huge exulcerating masses which eventually killed the mouse. The histological appearance of such a tumor is shown in Figs. 8 and 9.

The occasional regression of such tumors was the first observation which suggested to us that immune mechanisms might play a role in the postoncolytic period. The frequency of these tumors was variable. However, as a general rule we felt that oncolysis experiments performed with late A2G passages of EA tumor were more likely to lead to subcutaneous tumors than early passages. This was the only difference in behavior which seemed to have affected the EA line serially propagated in A2G mice. When oncolysis was performed in Sarcoma 180, the growth of solid tumors was only rarely observed. Apart from this unexplained difference in fre-

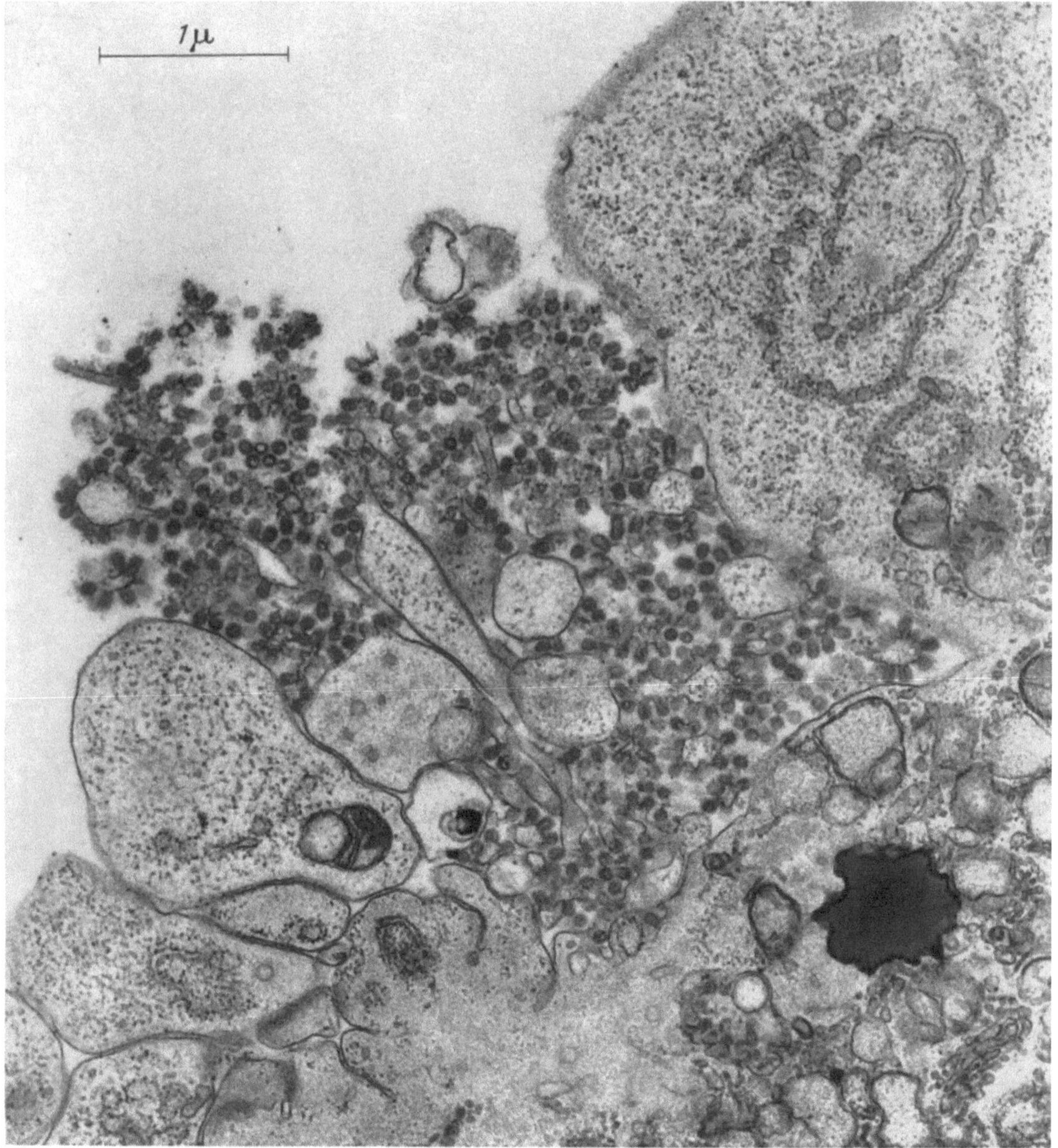

Fig. 6. Budding of WSA virus at the periphery of an Ehrlich ascites tumor cell, 36 hours after infection. The virus particles, mainly short rods, emerge from what seem to be altered microvilli

quency of subcutaneous tumors, oncolysis of Sarcoma 180 followed the same general pattern as oncolysis of EA, and the virus seemed to grow just as readily in both tumors.

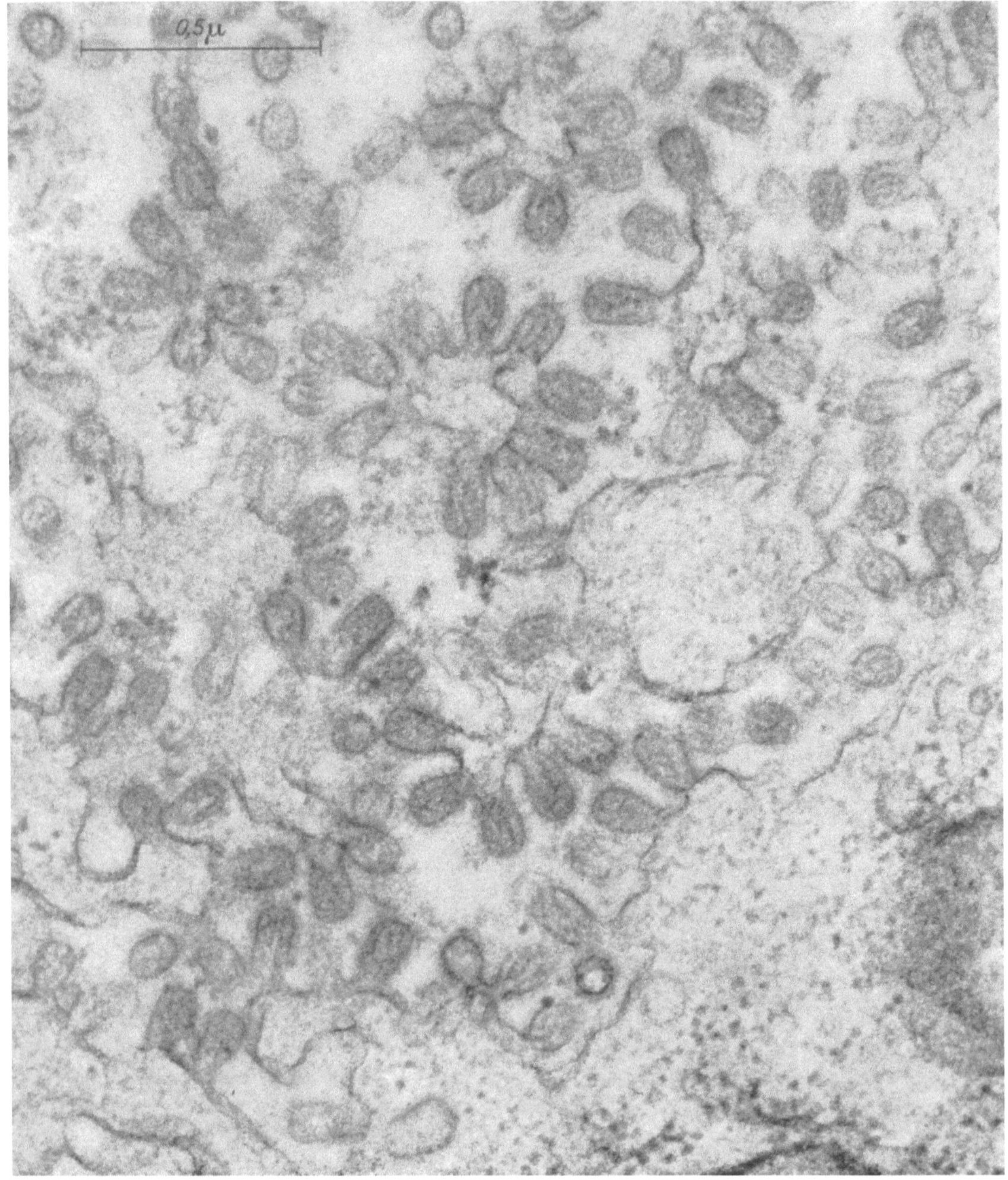

Fig. 7. Viral oncolysate produced by WSA virus in Ehrlich ascites tumor, 48 hours after infection. The periphery of a tumor cell occupies the lower right corner. Note continuity of cell membrane and viral membrane

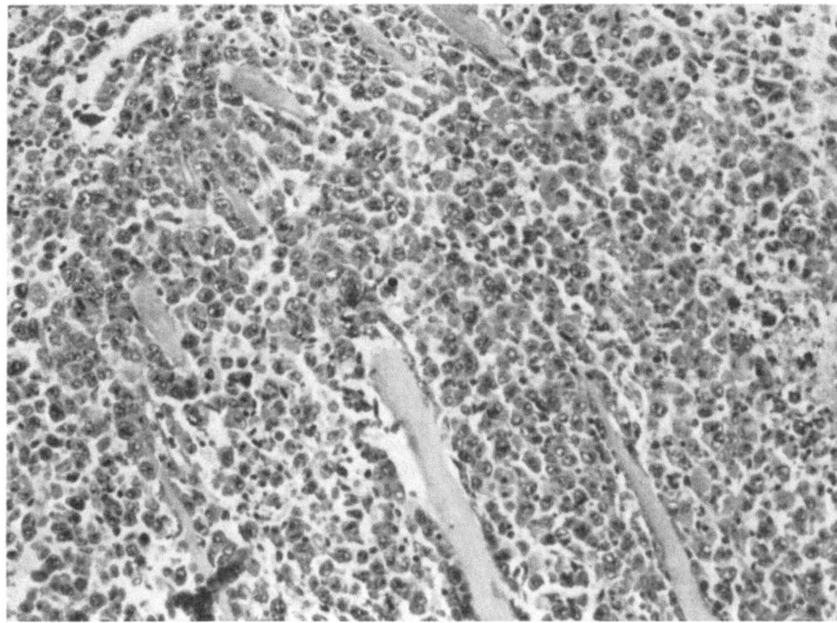

Fig. 8. Solid tumor growing at the site of the needle track of the original tumor inoculation, 2 weeks after oncolysis of Ehrlich ascites tumor by WSA virus. The tumor is infiltrating an abdominal muscle. HE stain, 200×

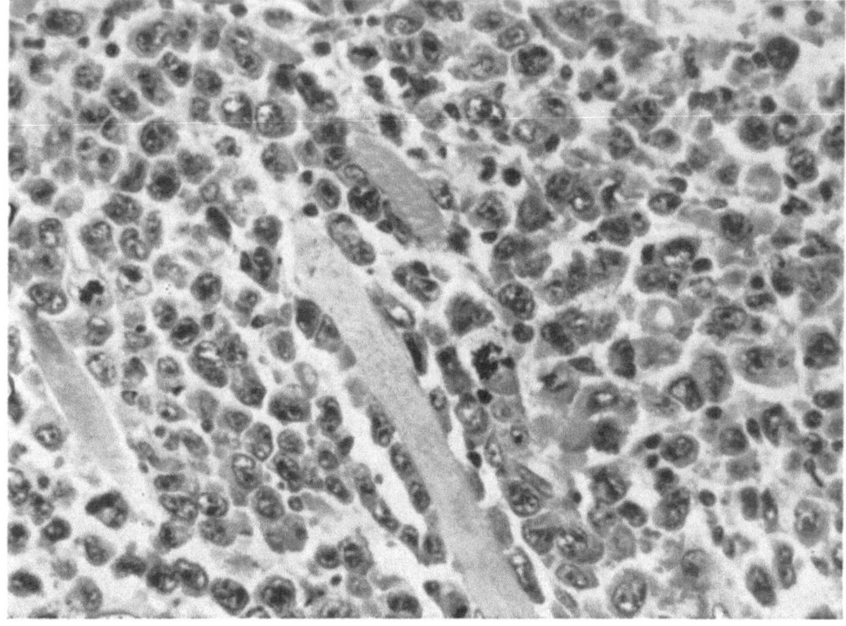

Fig. 9. Same as Fig. 8. 500×

2. The Immunity Induced by Oncolysis

a) Nature of the Immunity

As discussed earlier, evaluation of immunity levels in animals required quantitative information about the "virulence" of the disease inducing agent. Since the LD_{50}'s of the tumors used in our studies were close to 10 cells per mouse we found ourselves in possession of a most sensitive system to evaluate induced tumor immunity. However, our initial observations on postoncolytic immunity were so dramatic as to make such sensitivity unnecessary.

Over 50 A2G mice which had survived WSA oncolysis and were free of all detectable tumor were challenged with 10^6 viable EA cell (10^5 LD_{50}'s) from 3 weeks to 4 months after virus inoculation. None of these animals developed tumors while normal control animals uniformly succumbed to the tumor within 20 days. Such challenged "immune" mice were observed to be free of all tumor for at least 4 months. Some mice were kept more than a year without showing signs of relapse.

When the initial challenge dose was increased to 10^7 viable tumor cells, some mice died, but in a much delayed fashion. Other A2G mice survived but developed a transient ascites which reached its peak volume about the 14th to 20th day, then gradually became lax and finally regressed. Such transient ascitic fluids later proved to be rich sources of antibodies for immunochemical investigations.

The possibility was considered that this apparent "immune" phenomenon might have been due to the presence of residual WSA virus in postoncolytic mice. Such a possibility seemed, however, remote. It was known, for example, that WSA oncolysis did not occur in mice containing circulating anti-WSA antibodies (LINDENMANN, 1963). Circulating anti-WSA antibodies were present in high concentration as early as 8 days following WSA oncolysis. In addition, when mice were actively immunized with live egg-grown WSA and challenged with small numbers of tumor cells (1000 cells) 10 days after the primary virus inoculation, all mice invariably succumbed to the tumor. Routinely, however, post-oncolytic A2G mice were permitted a recuperative period of 30 days before they were subjected to tumor challenge. This was done mainly to allow those mice with subcutaneous tumors to show whether the subcutaneous growth would regress.

Since both cellular and humoral elements could have been contributing to the observed tumor immunity, we proceeded to investigate the phenomenon more closely. A test of the ability of spleen cells from immune A2G donors to confer protection on syngeneic non-immune recipients was performed (LINDENMANN, 1964 b). Spleen cells from A2G mice which had resisted rechallenge with 10^6 EA cells were harvested 5 weeks after tumor challenge. Syngeneic recipients received either 5×10^6 or 5×10^7 spleen cells or 0.5 ml of pooled serum from the same donors. Twenty-four hours later they were challenged with 10^4 viable EA cells (1000 LD_{50}'s). All mice pretreated with either cells or serum survived, whereas all control animals died of tumor. Serum protection proved to be more short-lived than cell protection, since all serum protected animals succumbed to a second tumor challenge of 10^4 cells 5 weeks later; all cell protected animals survived this second challenge. The long lasting effect of cellular transfer was evident even 17 weeks after the initial transfer when all recipients were challenged again, but this time with 10^6 EA cells. These results are summarized in Table 2. Thus, the observation that adoptive transfer of postoncolytic immunity was indeed possible, made such immunity similar to those involving allogeneic tumor grafts (MITCHISON, 1955).

Table 2. *Passive Protection of* A2G *Mice with Spleen Cells and Serum*

Pre-treatment	First challenge (10^4 EA cells i.p. 24 hours after transfer)	Second challenge (10^4 EA cells i.p. 5 weeks after transfer)	Third challenge (10^6 EA cells i.p. 17 weeks after transfer)
5×10^7 immune spleen cells i.p.	0/12 [a]	0/12	8/12
5×10^6 immune spleen cells i.p.	0/12	0/12	12/12 [b]
0.5 ml immune serum i.v. [c]	0/6	6/6	—
None	6/6	8/8	10/10 [d]

[a] No. of mice dying of ascites / No. of mice in each group.
[b] Mean survival time 22 days.
[c] Pooled serum from spleen cell donors.
[d] Mean survival time 17 days.

More surprising than this, however, was our finding that sera from immune animals could confer protection against tumor challenge. There has long been a controversy as to the role of humoral antibodies in homograft rejection and only recently has their possible role received renewed consideration (STETSON, 1963). We proceeded to investigate serum protection more thoroughly.

Serum harvested from 3 to 8 weeks after viral oncolysis followed by tumor challenge was effective in transfer of tumor immunity (LINDENMANN, 1964b). Normal A2G serum, normal ICR serum, ascitic fluid from A2G tumor-bearers, and mouse antisera directed against the oncolytic virus alone all failed to confer protection to A2G mice challenged with low doses of tumor (1000 cells). Serum from mice bearing 3 week old subcutaneous implants of the tumor likewise had no protective capacity.

Table 3. *Chessboard Titration of* A2G *Immune Serum in* A2G *Mice*

Serum dilution[a]	Challenge dose (No. of EA cells)		
	10^4	10^5	10^6
1:8	6/6 [b]	6/6	1/6
1:48	6/6	5/6	0/6
1:288	4/6	3/6	0/6
Normal A2G serum 1:4	0/6	0/6	0/6

[a] Final volume 0.5 ml. Serum and tumor cells inoculated together i.p.
[b] No. of mice surviving on day 28 / No. of mice in each group.

When the serum from a hyperimmune A2G mouse was titrated *in vivo* against varying numbers of tumor cells a definite pattern emerged. A typical experiment is presented in Table 3.

When large doses of antiserum were employed, protection against large numbers of tumor cells was possible. Some mice receiving small amounts of serum and high tumor doses failed to develop ascites but died of slowly growing subcutaneous or intraabdominal tumors. No instance of tumor enhancement was ever observed. Quite frequently we attempted to induce transient ascites formation by challenging immune A2G mice with 10^7 or 10^8 tumor cells. When ascites developed, the fluid was harvested between the 15th and 25th day post challenge. Although such fluids contained the protective factor, its titer was generally about 4 times lower than that of the corresponding serum. Yields of such ascites fluids varied from 12 to 30 ml per mouse.

We were delighted to find that postoncolytic A2G sera and ascites fluids produced a violent agglutination of tumor cells suspended in buffered saline. We have surveyed many fluids using this rather simple procedure and have found individual agglutination titers in sera of 1:100 to 1:5000 against 5×10^6 tumor cells. All postoncolytic sera produced so far in A2G mice have exhibited this property.

Ehrlich tumor cells could be heated to $56^0 C$ for over an hour without losing their agglutinability. Large numbers of tumor cells, either fresh or heated, were required for complete absorption of agglutinating antibody. We do not know if this reflects the low antigen concentration known to be present on the surface of nonspecific tumors (MÖLLER and MÖLLER, 1962) or poor binding efficiency between abundant antigenic sites and their corresponding antibody. In the few cytotoxicity tests performed by us, we have failed to detect cytotoxic antibodies in postoncolytic hyperimmune sera. This failure may be due to technical problems inherent in the test although the procedures have been those commonly employed in most laboratories concerned with cytotoxic phenomena (B. BENNETT, personal communication). Even alterations designed to increase the cytotoxic sensitivity of the basic test (BOYSE et al., 1962) have failed to yield evidence for any cytotoxic activity in postoncolytic immune sera. A good correlation has been shown to exist between cytotoxic sensitivity of normal and neoplastic mouse cells and concentration of alloantigenic receptor sites on the cell surface (MÖLLER and MÖLLER, 1962). It may be that the agglutinogen target on the Ehrlich cell is too sparsely distributed over the tumor surface for the antibody to act as a cytotoxin. Hemagglutination tests have failed to detect anti-H-2 specificity in A2G postoncolytic sera (J. PALM, personal communication).

Our early studies on the *in vivo* behavior of EA cells were concerned primarily with the ability of cells to initiate tumors following intraperitoneal residence in immune A2G mice. As late as 5 days after tumor inoculation mitoses were seen among tumor cells and only a fraction of less than 10 % of recoverable tumor cells stained with trypan blue. Tumor cells recovered from the peritoneal cavities of immune A2G mice up to the 4th day following challenge of the mice were able to induce tumor formation. We shall later describe experiments designed to examine host cell-tumor cell interactions in the presence and absence of specific immune globulin (see section e, p. 45).

A most interesting observation concerned the failure of A2G anti-EA serum to protect passively mice of strain ICR (LINDENMANN, 1964 b). At that time two possible hypotheses were set forth to explain this phenomenon. One of these suggested that ICR mice and the Ehrlich tumor might share a common cellular antigen. Thus, A2G anti-EA antibodies would be absorbed by normal mouse tissue before reaching the tumor during passive protection experiments with immune serum. The other hypothesis suggested that the ICR host cells involved in immune phagocytosis or clearance of the tumor were innately unable to "collaborate" with the A2G antibody which mediated such interactions. During the past several years we have accumulated evidence favoring the first hypothesis. This will be presented in sections e and g (p. 45 and 55).

b) Properties of the Protective Factor

Up to this point we have presented evidence that sera from postoncolytic A2G mice contained a factor which could confer passive protection to syngeneic mice against Ehrlich tumor. We suspected that this factor was an antibody and assessed its nature with the help of several of the tools commonly employed in immunochemistry.

Results of sucrose gradient zone sedimentation and column electrophoresis, which showed a good correlation between agglutinin titers of the fractions and protective potency, have been published previously (LINDENMANN, 1964 b). A number of additional fractionations have been performed since and will be briefly summarized. Thus, electrophoresis of postoncolytic serum in a Pevikon block showed both agglutinin and protective activity in the zones corresponding to the gamma globulin region. Agglutinating and protective activity were eluted from DEAE cellulose by .04 to .08 M phosphate buffer (pH 7.9). Gel filtration of postoncolytic serum on a column of Sephadex G-200 revealed the presence of agglutinating and protective activity in the central peak, the first and the third peak being inactive. All these data suggested that the protective factor and the agglutinin were antibodies of the 7S or IgG immunoglobulin class. Since all sera analyzed by the above procedures were from hyperimmune animals which had been subjected to at least one tumor challenge, the possibility remains that early antibodies may be different.

c) The ε-Alloantigen

The in *vitro* agglutination assay for anti-EA antibody discussed in the last section allowed us to screen postoncolytic sera quite rapidly for the presence or absence of agglutinin. Since the agglutinogen-agglutinin reaction most probably represented a non H-2 antigen-antibody union we were interested in the nature of the agglutinogen and other antigens found in the Ehrlich tumor cells. Mouse cellular alloantigens are generally detected by techniques such as cytotoxicity, leukocyte agglutination, hemagglutination, hemagglutination-inhibition, immunofluorescence, induction of tumor homograft enhancement or accelerated homograft rejection. Mouse heteroantigens of cellular origin have been detected using gel-diffusion techniques with rabbit antibodies (BOYLE et al., 1963), but mouse cellular alloantigens have not been detectable by this procedure using mouse alloantibody (D.A.L. DAVIES, personal communication).

Our early attempts to detect soluble antigens in EA cells using A2G hyperimmune serum in gel diffusion assays against tumor cell extracts all proved to be futile. We were about to abandon this series of experiments when an immune A2G ascites fluid was discovered which precipitated in gel diffusion assays with lysates of the Ehrlich tumor (LINDENMANN and KLEIN, 1964). When this fluid (no. 24) was tested in Ouchterlony type double diffusion gel precipitation tests against an aqueous extract of Ehrlich tumor cells, a single precipitation line formed between the two wells. We called the antigen thus detectable in the lysate, ε.

When aqueous extracts of the Krebs-2 and Sarcoma 180 tumors were tested against fluid no. 24 they gave reactions identical to those produced by the Ehrlich tumor. Extracts from the strain specific Sarcoma I ascites tumor showed no precipitation under the same conditions. These reactions are presented in Fig. 10.

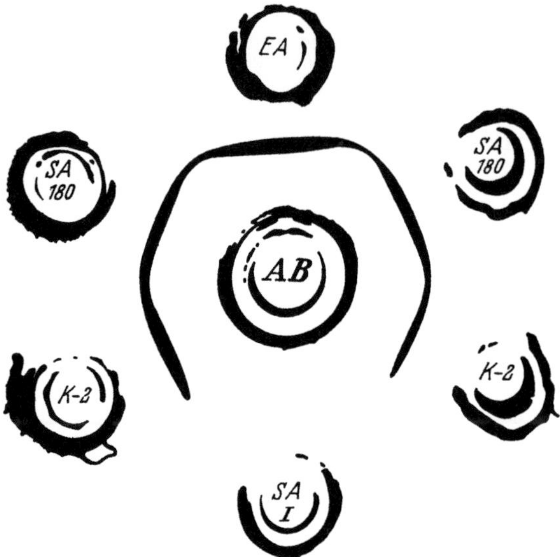

Fig. 10. Gel diffusion analysis of postoncolytic A2G antiserum, aqueous extracts from 3 nonspecific tumors and one strain specific tumor indigenous to strain A. Center well contains A2G antiserum No. 24. Peripheral wells contain aqueous extracts of mouse tumor cells prepared as indicated in the text. Precipitin lines formed by antibody reacting with Ehrlich, Krebs-2, and Sarcoma 180 extracts coalesce, indicating a reaction of identity. Note lack of reaction between Sarcoma I (specific for strain A mice) extract and A2G antibody

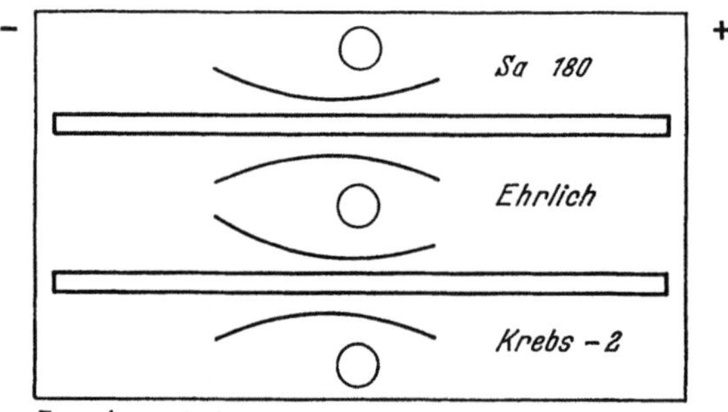

Fig. 11. Immuno-electrophoresis of precipitating antigen in 3 tumor extracts. Centrifuged (15,000 rpm, 30 min.) extracts of the 3 tumors, Sarcoma 180, Ehrlich ascites, and Krebs-2, were equilibrated by dialysis against pH 8.6 Veronal buffer before being placed in their respective wells. The troughs all contain A2G alloantibody No. 24

Immunoelectrophoresis of the ε-alloantigen from the 3 nonspecific tumors against no. 24 fluid revealed that they had quite similar electrophoretic properties (Fig. 11).

We decided to see if the ε-alloantigen could be detected in the normal organs of various inbred strains of mice. The preparation of water soluble antigen from these strains was accomplished in a variety of ways. These are described in Fig. 12.

Chloroform extraction was a very effective purification step which removed much non-reactive material from such lysates without affecting the stability, yield, or activity of ε. The organs extracted in this way included liver, spleen, pancreas, brain, kidney and heart. In all tests reported a given strain either possessed the ε-antigen

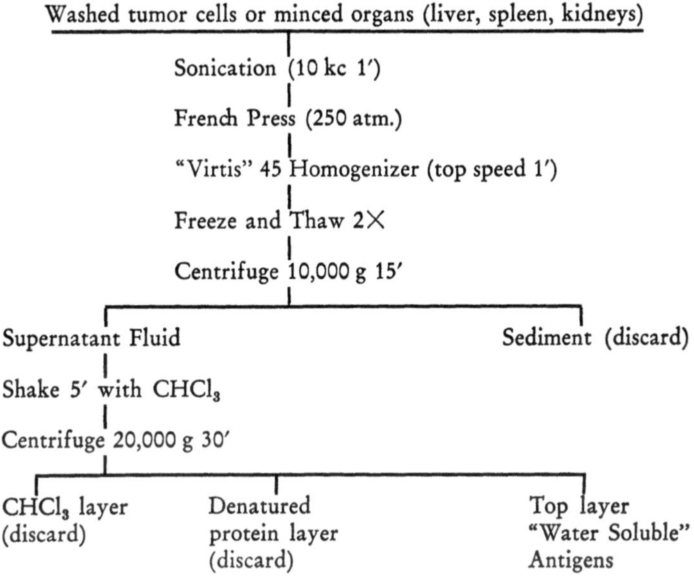

Fig. 12. Usual methods for the preparation of water soluble antigens from normal mouse organs or mouse tumors. Any one of the 3 cell breakage procedures mentioned in the flow sheet worked equally well. Thus, *either* sonication, passage through the French press, or homogenization in a Virtis homogenizer could be used. The remaining extraction steps shown on the flow sheet were applied sequentially

in all organs tested or lacked it completely in these same tissues. We never observed that some organs contained ε and others lacked ε in the same animal. The concentration of ε, however, varied from organ to organ. Thus, liver and spleen were somewhat richer in the antigen than brain. Normal mouse serum from all strains tested failed to precipitate with no. 24 fluid. Whole ICR embryos of 15 days gestation contained the antigen. Table 4 summarizes our findings to date on the distribution of the ε antigen in various mouse strains and in some mouse tumors.

There is no obvious relationship of the ε-antigen to the strong H-2 locus of the mouse. For example, strain A mice which are H-2ª lack ε whereas B10.A mice, likewise H-2ª and congenic with C57BL/10, contain ε. In addition, H-2ᵏ is represented in mice which have ε (C58/J) and in mice which lack ε (C₃H). Several of the strains lacking ε are closely related. Thus, A2G and A are of similar derivation, as are AKR and RF, and CBA and C3H. All these were derived at some time from Bagg albino mice (STAATS, 1964).

The strain distribution of the ε-alloantigen made it likely that its presence or absence was under genetic control. Preliminary analysis of F₁ offspring from crosses where only one of the parents contained the antigen revealed that such mice contained one half as much ε as homozygous ε positive animals. Table 5 shows that segregation occurred when F_1 males were backcrossed to ε negative females. It should be pointed out that the use of A2G mice instead of A mice as the backcross parent does not invalidate this test. We have already discussed the similarities of these two strains. This result suggests that ε is controlled by a single dominant gene in inbred mice.

Table 4. *Distribution of ε-antigen Among Various Strains of Mice and Four Mouse Tumors* [a]

ε present		ε absent
BaB	Multiplex [b]	A2G
BALB/cJ	PL/J	A/J
BUA	RIII/J	A/HeJ
B10.A/Sn [c]	S/Gw	AKR/J
C57BL/6J	SJL/J	AL/Ks
C57BL/10J	ST/J	CBA/J
C57BR/cdJ	SWR/J	C3H/HeJ
C57L/J	Z/Gw	C3HeB/FeJ
C58/J	129/J	C3H.K/Sn [d]
DBA/1J	B6D2F1/J	LG
DBA/2J	B6AF1/J [e]	RF/J
DD/He	B6A2F1/K [e]	Sa I tumor
E/Gw	Ehrlich tumor	
ICR [f]	Krebs-2 tumor	
MA/J	Sa 180 tumor	

    [a] Aqueous organ or tumor extracts were assayed in an immunodiffusion test against A2G alloantibody No. 24.
    [b] Received from Dr. M. E. WALLACE.
    [c] H—2ᵃ on C57BL/10 genetic background.
    [d] H—1ᵇ on C3H genetic background.
    [e] Weaker reactions.
    [f] Non-inbred.

Table 5. *Inheritance of ε-antigen in Mice*

Mice	No. tested	No. ε-positive	No. ε-negative
A/J	10	0	10
A2G	many	0	all
C57BL/6J	10	10	0
B6AF1 [a]	10	10	0
B6AF1×A2G [b]	98	47 [c]	51 [c]

    [a] (A×C57BL/6)F1.
    [b] Cross of B6AF1 males with A2G females.
    [c] $p=0.5$—0.7 under the assumption of a single dominant gene.

Congenic resistant inbred mouse strains kindly supplied by Dr. G. D. Snell enabled us to test the relationship between the ε-alloantigen and 9 of the 11 known autosomal histocompatibility loci of the mouse. Two loci, H-5 and H-6 (AMOS et al., 1963), which have only recently been reported, could not be tested by this procedure, since congenic strains involving these loci are unavailable (G. D. Snell, personal communication). Our observation that C57BL/10 mice possessed ε formed the basis of this experiment. Congenic resistant strains differing from each other at single histocompatibility loci and all derived from C57BL/10 inbred partners had been developed (SNELL, 1958). Since the inbred partner C57BL/10 contained ε the effect of changes at each of 9 histocompatibility loci on the expression of ε could be examined. Table 6 presents the results of our tests. It is clear that substitutions at each of the 9 loci were without effect on ε.

Table 6. *Independence of the ε-alloantigen Locus from Nine Major Histocompatibility Loci*

Mouse strain	Allele present at:									ε
	H-1	H-2	H-3	H-4	H-7	H-8	H-9	H-10	H-11	
C57BL/10ScSn [a]	c	b	a	a	a	a	a	a	a	+[b]
B10.BY	*d*	b	a	a	a	a	a	a	a	+
B10.D2	c	*d*	a	a	a	a	a	a	a	+
B10.LP	c	b	*b*	a	a	a	a	a	a	+
B10.129 (21M)	c	b	a	*b*	a	a	a	a	a	+
B10.C (47N)	c	b	a	a	*b*	a	a	a	a	+
B10.D2 (57N)	c	b	a	a	a	*b*	a	a	a	+
B10.C (45N)	c	b	a	a	a	a	*b*	a	a	+
B10.129 (9M)	c	b	a	a	a	a	a	*b*	a	+
B10.129 (10M)	c	b	a	a	a	a	a	a	*b*	+

[a] Inbred partner for all congenic derivatives used in this test.

[b] ε was assayed in aqueous organ extracts of individual mice in gel diffusion tests with anti-ε alloantibody. + indicates a positive precipitation reaction.

This was a most interesting finding because it suggested that ε might be an extremely "weak" cellular antigen. Rejection of skin grafts across the H-11 locus, for example, requires about 100 days (SNELL, 1965). If ε really is a weak histocompatibility factor of the mouse then it must be assumed that viral oncolysis has enormously enhanced its immunogenicity. Since the discovery of anti-ε fluid no. 24, we have found that most postoncolytic A2G mice eventually develop the anti ε precipitin. One to 3 days after oncolysis ε is readily detected in the serum of A2G mice (KLEIN and LINDENMANN, unpublished). This is probably the result of tumor cell destruction by the virus. By the 8th day following oncolysis anti-EA agglutinin appears in the circulation of such mice. We have no convincing evidence, however, that ε and the agglutinogen are the same.

Our preliminary findings on the biochemical properties of the ε antigen are summarized in Table 7.

The antigen is stable under a variety of conditions. For example, it may be frozen at $-15\,^{\circ}$C and thawed for a practically unlimited number of cycles. Tumor cells or tissues containing ε may be stored for many days at 4 °C before the antigen is extracted from them. Such storage in no way affects the final yield of the antigen from these cells. This may mean that ε is relatively unaffected by most of the intracellular degradative enzymes present in cells containing the antigen under the above conditions. Extraction of the antigen by means of sonication must break open many lysosomes and yet this procedure does not affect the final yield.

The fact that chloroform extraction left ε unaffected in the aqueous phase might mean that lipids were either absent from or unnecessary for the immunochemical reactivity of the molecule. This point will require clarification in the future, but if it is true then it most probably means that ε is different from the lipoproteins isolated from the H-2 antigenic complex of the mouse. Although water-soluble antigenic materials with H-2 specificity have been reported, these have been only partially characterized (KAHAN, 1965; HAUGHTON, 1965).

Enzyme degradation studies revealed that the antigen probably was devoid of nucleic acids. The failure of neuraminidase to destroy the ability of ε to precipitate with antibody argued against involvement of neuraminic acid containing moieties

Table 7. *Properties of the ε-alloantigen*

Treatment of ε-alloantigen[a]	Precipitation with A2G anti-ε after treatment
1. *pH*	
2—3 for 24 hours at $+4°$ C	—
4—10 for 24 hours at $+4°$ C	+
2. *Temperature*	
40—60° C for 80 min. at pH 7.2	+
70° C for 80 min. at pH 7.2	—
3. *Enzymes and periodate*	
DNAase (20 µg)	+
RNAase (25 µg)	+
Neuraminidase (0.25 µmolar units)	+
Trypsin (100 µg)	—
Trypsin + soy bean trypsin inhibitor	+
$NaIO_4$ (meta) 0.01 M	—
4. *Storage, dialysis*	
Storage of whole ε-positive cells for 9 days at $+4°$ C followed by extraction of ε	+
Freezing and thawing 50 times	+
Lyophilization and reconstitution	+
Dialysis against running tap water, 48 hours	+
5. *Extraction and precipitation*	
$CHCl_3$ 5 times, test aqueous phase	+
Sonication 10 Kc for 10 min. at $+4°$ C	+
$(NH_4)_2SO_4$: 0.5 saturated supernatant	+
0.7 saturated supernatant	—
0.7 saturated precipitate	+
Centrifugation 105,000 g 60 min. supernatant	+

[a] Crude lysate of $4\times$ washed Ehrlich ascites cells.

within the active antigenic site of the molecule. This finding was most interesting since the same concentration of enzyme could destroy the receptors for WSA virus on fowl erythrocytes and the receptors for reovirus type 3 on human type 0 erythrocytes. Although the neuraminidase activity of the neurotropic WSA virus is peculiar and that of the reovirus ill-defined, these enzymes may play some role in the liberation of immunogenic molecules from virus-infected tumor cells. We shall see later that neuraminidase containing preparations could effect active immunization of tumor-bearing A2G mice (see section h, p. 63).

Destruction of ε occurred when the antigen was treated with trypsin. This experiment was carried out using both crude tumor cell lysates and partially purified antigen with no difference being observed. Crystalline soybean trypsin inhibitor was capable of preventing the destruction of ε by trypsin. These observations in conjunction with the finding that periodate oxidation also effected destruction of ε, suggested that the antigen might be a glycoprotein.

High speed centrifugation of ε-positive tumor cell lysates failed to sediment the antigen. This suggested that an estimate of the molecular weight of ε might be achieved by gel filtration (ANDREWS, 1964). This relatively simple procedure, however, required that several assumptions be made about the molecule under consideration: Globular configuration in solution and low carbohydrate content (ANDREWS, 1965). The results of such an experiment are shown in Fig. 13.

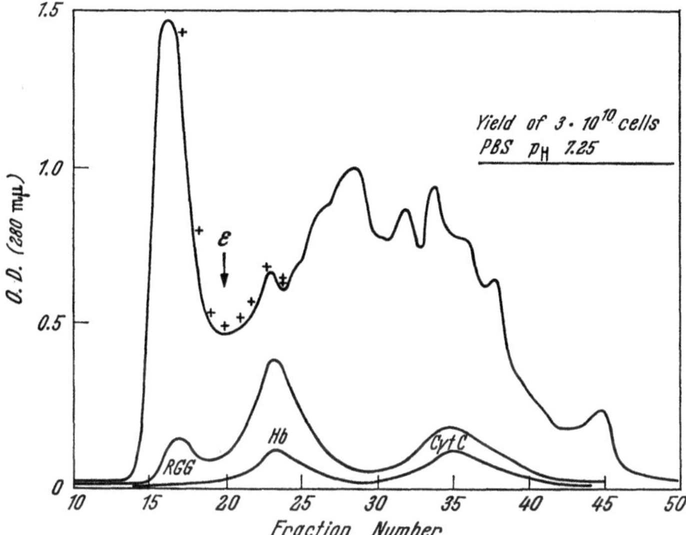

Fig. 13. Fractionation of an extract of Ehrlich ascites tumor cells on Sephadex G-100. Five ml of an extract from 3×10^{10} EA cells containing 2 grams of protein were applied to a column 2.5×50 cm. Preliminary tests had indicated that ε antigen could still be detected at 1 : 40 dilution. Fractions of 5 ml were eluted with phosphate buffered saline (pH 7.2) and were assayed in gel-diffusion tests with A2G anti-ε alloantibody for the presence or absence of precipitating antigen. The column employed was first calibrated by chromatography of a mixture containing rabbit gamma-globulin, human hemoglobin, and horse cytochrome c, each at a concentration of 10 mg/ml. The location of the rabbit gamma-globulin was confirmed with specific goat antiserum. The lowest curve represents absorption at 540 mμ. A plot of elution volume versus log. of the molecular weight of the markers yields an estimate of 80,000 for the molecular weight of the ε-alloantigen

Since the column had been pre-calibrated with known molecular weight markers, we were able to arrive at an estimate of 80 000 for the molecular weight of the ε-alloantigen. This estimate, however, was made with full awareness of the assumptions made above. ε was thus considerably smaller than the *H-2* component described by KAHAN (1965), who inferred a molecular weight of 200 000 for his H-2 specific moiety.

The G-100 fractions containing ε were pooled and concentrated. This pool was then fractionated by chromatography on DEAE cellulose. Fig. 14 shows the result of this experiment.

When we similarly chromatographed an ε-containing *viral* oncolysate of ε-positive cells, the ε antigen was eluted from the column at the same salt concentrations. This suggested that the antigen had the same charge properties when released from cells by physical lysis or by viral lysis. This impression has been confirmed by immunoelectrophoresis.

A2G mice lacked the ε-alloantigen as detected in immunoprecipitation tests with A2G immune serum. We considered the possibility that such mice might possess an allotype of ε (KLEIN and LINDENMANN, 1965). If this were true then an anti-ε antibody raised in A2G mice would be directed against only those amino acid sequences which differentiate the ε allotypes within the murine species (CINADER and

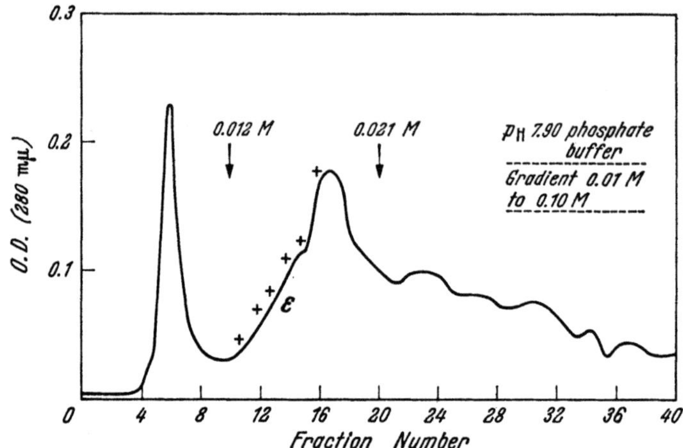

Fig. 14. Ion exchange chromatography of Ehrlich ascites tumor cell extract on DEAE cellulose. Fractions No. 18 to 22 from the Sephadex G-100 separation shown in Fig. 13 were pooled and concentrated to 44 mg protein/ml. 2.2 ml of this preparation were applied to a 1.2×10 cm column of DEAE cellulose and eluted with a linear concentration gradient (0.01 M NaCl to 0.10 M NaCl in pH 7.9 phosphate buffer). Fractions of 2 ml were collected. ε was assayed by gel diffusion tests with A2G anti-ε alloantibody

Table 8. *Distribution of ε-like Antigen Among Various Species* [a]

Human liver	4/4[b]	Chick	2/2
HeLa cells	1/1	Chick embryo	2/2
Marmoset liver	1/1	Duck	1/1
Pony spleen [c]	?/1	Gopher turtle	1/1
Calf thymus	6/6	Cottonmouth snake	0/1
Sheep liver	1/1	Frog	0/1
Rabbit liver	3/3	Smelt	0/1
Hamster liver	4/4	Shrimp	0/1
Guinea pig liver	1/1	Clam	0/1
Rat liver	1/1	Pneumoc. SSS I [d]	0/1
		Salm. O antigen [e]	0/1

[a] Organ or whole animal extracts were assayed in gel-diffusion tests with A2G anti-ε antibody. For more exact definition of animals used, see KLEIN and LINDENMANN (1965).

[b] No. positive / No. tested.

[c] Equivocal result.

[d] Pneumococcal capsular polysaccharide type I.

[e] O antigen from Salmonella typhimurium.

DUBISKI, 1964). This would mean that the reactivity of such an A2G anti-ε antibody with xenogeneic ε molecules would be limited to closely related species. On the other hand, if A2G mice lacked entirely a molecule related to ε, we would expect the antibody to react with ε-like molecules from many xenogeneic sources. These alternatives were tested by preparing aqueous extracts of organs and whole organisms from various species and testing them in gel-diffusion assays against A2G anti-ε antibody. Table 8 shows the results of these tests.

Most immunoprecipitation patterns thus obtained were as clear as in the mouse systems previously described. Where a line of precipitation was observed it could be shown to coalesce with the line formed against an ε-positive murine extract. Reactions obtained with pony lymph node extracts and cow liver were not clear-cut. Slight differences in the electrophoretic properties were noted in these ε-like moieties when compared to ε of murine origin. These results suggested that the A2G mouse does not contain an ε-allotype in its tissues but lacks a corresponding substance entirely [2]. All ε-negative mouse strains may not, however, behave in the same manner. Future experiments may yet reveal ε allotypes among some of them. The distribution of the ε-alloantigen made it highly unlikely that it was related to the classical Forssman antigen (R. NELSON, personal communication). For example, it was present in sheep liver which lacks the Forssman antigen, but absent from sheep erythrocytes which contain the Forssman antigen.

We know little about the exact cellular localization of the ε-alloantigen. We do know, however, that anti-ε antibody can be removed from A2G serum with Ehrlich tumor cells. This suggests that the antigen is either on or near the surface of such cells. Its presence does not seem to confer any growth predilection on tumors carrying it. Thus, EA cells which contain the antigen grew equally well in A2G mice which lack ε and in ICR mice which contain it. After 130 passages in A2G mice, EA tumor cells contained levels of ε similar to those found in a parallel line of the tumor passed exclusively in ICR mice. It seems that little selective pressure was exerted, therefore, against cells possessing ε during growth in mice devoid of this antigen.

The presence or absence of ε seemed to be independent of myxovirus resistance in inbred mouse strains (LINDENMANN and KLEIN, 1966). The role of ε in the economy of cells containing it, its relationship to the agglutinogen discussed earlier, and its role in the induction of postoncolytic tumor immunity are all questions of great interest. Some of our preliminary findings will be discussed in later sections. It must be pointed out that a least 2 other cellular alloantigens have been observed using postoncolytic A2G serum in gel diffusion assays. Antibodies to these appeared quite irregularly so that we have very small quantities of alloantibody to these antigens. We only mention this fact to emphasize the usefulness of viral oncolysis for uncovering alloantigenic specificities which might otherwise be extremely difficult to detect.

d) Cross Protection Between Nonspecific Tumors

Postoncolytic immunity to rechallenge with the Ehrlich tumor was described previously. When A2G mice which had resisted challenge with this tumor were rechallenged with 1000 LD_{50}'s of either Krebs-2 or Sarcoma 180 ascites cells they failed to develop tumors. It must be remembered that the LD_{50} of all 3 tumors was under 100 cells in A2G mice. A2G mice which had just recuperated from viral oncolysis of the Ehrlich tumor likewise failed to develop tumors when given a primary challenge of either K-2 or Sa 180. All such mice survived challenge with 10^4 K-2 cells, but none survived challenge with 10^6 K-2 cells. However, mice challenged

---

[2] Note added in proof: The term "eniotype" has recently been proposed for this state of affairs (CINADER, B., S. DUBISKI, and A. C. WARDLAW: Allotypy and eniotypy. Nature (Lond.) **210**, 1291 (1966)).

with 10^4 K-2 cells a first time were resistant to rechallenge with 10^6 K-2 cells several weeks later. When the primary challenge was 10^4 or 10^6 Sa 180 cells all mice survived. Rechallenge with 10^7 Sa 180 cells several weeks after a first challenge with 10^6 Sa 180 cells failed to induce tumors. It seemed that active immunity to Sa 180 was of similar magnitude to that observed with the Ehrlich tumor. Cross immunity to K-2 seemed less pronounced (LINDENMANN and KLEIN, 1965). Challenge with any one of the three tumors seemed to produce a booster effect against all others.

We have already discussed the fact that all three tumors, K-2, EA, and Sa 180 contained the ε-alloantigen. We soon found that A2G anti-EA postoncolytic sera would agglutinate both K-2 and Sa 180 tumor cells. Sa 180 cells were agglutinated to titers quite comparable to those of Ehrlich cells. However, at times we had difficulties with suspensions of K-2 cells which showed in controls high levels of spontaneous agglutination. In those instances where this difficulty was not encountered, titers obtained with K-2 and EA cell suspensions were identical within a four-fold range. A comparison of the ability of K-2 and EA cells to absorb the agglutinating antibody from A2G serum revealed that K-2 cells were less efficient than comparable numbers of EA cells (LINDENMANN and KLEIN, 1965).

A series of passive protection experiments were performed involving the transfer of immunity to K-2 and Sa 180 using A2G anti-EA sera. The results of a typical experiment are described in Table 9.

Table 9. *Passive Protection of A2G Mice with post-oncolytic Serum (A2G anti-EA) against, EA, K-2 and Sa 180 Ascites Tumors*

Challenge dose (No. of cells)	Control mice			Serum protected mice		
	EA	K-2	Sa 180	EA [a]	K-2 [a]	Sa 180 [b]
25	10/10 [c]	10/10	n. d. [d]	0/10	4/10	n. d.
250	10/10	10/10	n. d.	0/10	6/10	n. d.
500	10/10	n. d.	10/10	0/10	n. d.	0/10
2500	10/10	10/10	n. d.	0/10	10/10	n. d.
5000	10/10	n. d.	10/10	0/10	n. d.	0/10
25,000	10/10	10/10	n. d.	5/10	10/10	n. d.
50,000	n. d.	n. d.	n. d.	n. d.	n. d.	0/10
500,000	n. d.	n. d.	n. d.	n. d.	n. d.	2/10

[a] 0.02 ml of serum No. 4 mixed with tumor inoculum and injected intraperitoneally.
[b] 0.02 ml of serum No. 8 mixed with tumor inoculum and injected intraperitoneally.
[c] No. of mice dying of ascites / No. of mice in each group.
[d] n. d. = not done.

With Sa 180 and EA (see above) the levels of protection attained were quite similar. However, the same amount of immune serum seemed to protect mice against 100 to 1000 times fewer K-2 cells than EA cells. Indeed, the protection afforded against K-2 may seem borderline. We have recently, however, obtained sera which protected A2G mice against 5000 K-2 cells when used in 0.02 ml amounts.

Our finding that antigenic similarities existed among several nonspecific tumors was in agreement with an earlier report on cross-protection of mice in a different viral oncolysis system (KOPROWSKI et al., 1957). We considered the possibility that the observed similarities might indeed be insignificant, since the three tumors used might be identical or of common derivation. As we have said previously the possible identity of hypotetraploid lines of the Ehrlich tumor and the Krebs-2 tumor has been argued by some. The Sa 180 tumor has never been suspected of identity with EA or K-2. In fact, our cross-protection data reveal more of a similarity between EA and Sa 180 than between EA and K-2. We have already pointed out that the antigenic similarities observed were present when tumor cells were examined directly from the hosts in which they came to us. We are thus quite confident that they were not the result of the confusion of tumors during passages in our laboratories.

e) Passive Protection of Syngeneic and Allogeneic Mice with A2G Immune Serum

The failure of A2G anti-EA immune serum to protect passively ICR mice has been a most perplexing finding. We have pursued several different lines of investigation in an attempt to arrive at some understanding of this phenomenon. Some of these have been reported elsewhere (KLEIN and LINDENMANN, 1965) and others represent experiments currently in progress in our laboratories.

We first considered the possibility that the protective antibody in postoncolytic A2G serum was identical with the anti-ε precipitin. If this were true, we reasoned that perhaps all mice posessing the ε-alloantigen would not be passively protectable since the protective antibody would be neutralized by the ε component of normal tissues. On the other hand, one would expect all mouse strains lacking ε to be passively protectable.

A preliminary test was performed in which the protective power of an A2G antiserum was assessed in syngeneic A2G mice. At a dilution of 1:10, 0.5 ml of this serum afforded complete protection against 50 000 EA cells to 100 % of A2G mice. In passive protection tests involving other strains of mice 0.5 ml of a 1:5 dilution of this antiserum was employed per mouse against a challenge dose of 50 000 EA cells. Mice surviving 30 days were considered protected if they showed no gross evidence of ascitic or subcutaneous tumor. All control mice of all strains employed were invariably dead of tumor by that time. Results of such tests on ε-containing strains are shown in Table 10, those performed on ε-lacking strains are shown in Table 11.

With the exception of two strains (PL and RIII) all ε containing strains were non-protectable under the conditions just described. Of those strains lacking ε four were clearly protectable and two were clearly non-protectable (RF and LG). One strain (AKR) has consistently yielded intermediate results in these tests just as have PL and RIII above. The two ε-lacking strains which were non-protectable could perhaps contain an ε allotype in their tissues capable of neutralizing the protective A2G antibody. But what then can we say about those ε-containing mice which to some degree at least proved to be protectable? Much further work remains to be done before this question can be settled. As we shall see later antibody seems to be an essential component in the immunity sequence. The role of complement components may be quite important. However, we cannot attribute failure to achieve passive protection in some strains to a lack of a complement component in their circulation (CINADER et al., 1964). In addition we have not been able to explain failure of passive protection by assuming that some strains synthesize an anti-A2G antibody when the A2G globulin is passively administered to them. This assumption is not supported by available data concerning the distribution of immunoglobulin allotypes in inbred strains of mice (HERZENBERG et al., 1965).

We have begun a series of experiments offering a more direct approach to the problem of non-protectability. While this work is very preliminary we feel it merits discussion at this point. Groups of A2G and ICR mice were inoculated with 5×10^5

Table 10. *Passive Protection of Various Mouse Strains with* A2G *anti-EA Serum. A. Mouse Strains Containing the ε-antigen*

Mouse strain	Control (no serum)[a]	Serum protected[b]
BALB/cJ	0/5 [c]	0/5
C58/J	0/5	0/5
DBA/1J	0/5	0/5
DBA/2J	0/5	0/5
ICR (non-inbred)	0/10	0/10
MA/J	0/5	0/5
PL/J	0/5	1/5
RIII/J	0/11	3/11
ST/J	0/5	0/5
SWR/J	0/5	0/5
129/J	0/5	0/5
CAF1 (BALB/cJ×A/J)	0/5	0/5
C3D2F1 (C3H/HeJ×DBA/2J)	0/5	0/5

[a] 50,000 washed EA cells injected intraperitoneally.

[b] 50,000 washed EA cells injected together with 0.5 ml of a 1:5 dilution of A2G anti-EA serum intraperitoneally.

[c] No. of mice protected / No. of mice in each group. Final readings on day 30.

Table 11. *Passive Protection of Various Mouse Strains with A2G anti-EA Serum. B. Mouse Strains Lacking the ε-antigen*

Mouse strain	Control (no serum)[a]	Serum protected[b]
A2G	0/10 [c]	10/10
A/J	0/5	5/5
AKR/J	0/11	2/11
C3H/HeJ	0/5	5/5
CBA/J	0/5	5/5
LG	0/4	0/4
RF/J	0/11	0/11

[a] 50,000 washed EA cells injected intraperitoneally.

[b] 50,000 washed EA cells injected together with 0,5 ml of a 1:5 dilution of A2G anti-EA serum intraperitoneally.

[c] No. of mice protected / No. of mice in each group. Final reading on day 30.

EA cells and either normal A2G serum or postoncolytic A2G anti-EA immune serum. At 1, 9, 24, 44 and 80 hours post inoculation 3 animals from each group were exsanguinated. Serum was obtained from individual mice and tested in slide agglutination tests for its tumor agglutination titer. The peritoneal cavities of all mice were washed out with buffered saline and determinations of the total number of tumor cells per mouse were made. In addition, smears of individual peritoneal exudates were fixed, and stained with Giemsa. These smears were then examined microscopically and differential counts were performed to ascertain the % of tumor cells in intimate contact with host cells (polymorphonuclear leucocytes and macrophages). This experiment is described in Figures 15a, 15b and 15c.

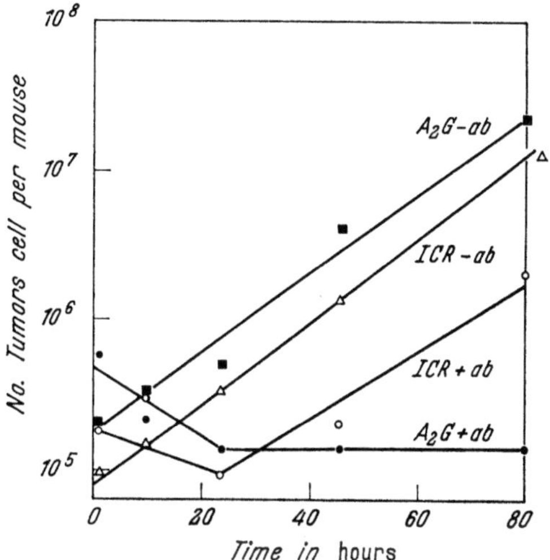

Fig. 15a. Growth of Ehrlich ascites tumor in passively immunized and in control A2G and ICR mice. Each point represents the average of the total tumor cell count from 3 mice. Zero hour points represent average initial inoculum per group of animals. Passively immunized mice received 3,000 "agglutinating units" (0.6 ml of a serum with a tumor agglutination titer of 1 : 5,000) of an A2G anti-EA serum at 0 hour with the tumor cell inoculum

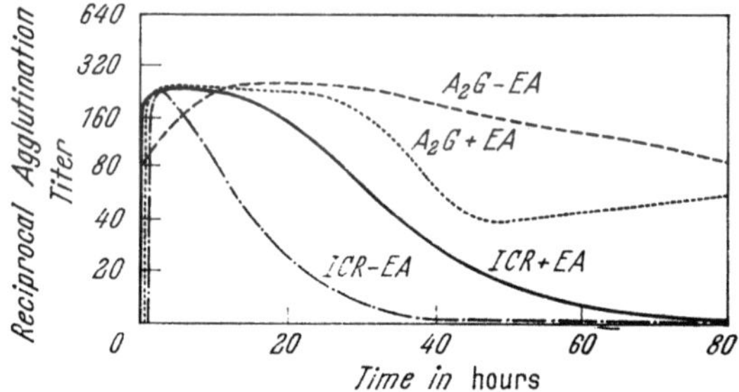

Fig. 15b. Fate of A2G anti-EA antibody in tumor-bearing and tumor-free A2G and ICR mice. The tumor-bearing groups represented are the same as in Fig. 15a. Serum was harvested from individual mice prior to tumor cell counting (Fig. 15a) at 1, 9, 24. 44 and 80 hours and assayed for tumor agglutination titer by quantitative slide tests. Agglutination titers of 3 individual mice were averaged at each time interval for each group

Figure 15a shows the growth patterns of the Ehrlich tumor in ICR and A2G mice with and without postoncolytic A2G anti-EA immune serum. The growth rate of the tumor was strikingly similar in both A2G and ICR mice not treated with serum. In A2G and ICR mice receiving immune serum, however, the growth of the tumor appeared to be inhibited to the same extent for the first 24 hours. After this time the tumor resumed rapid growth in ICR animals, whereas tumor growth continued to be suppressed in A2G mice. We have mentioned previously that viable tumor cells were readily recoverable from peritoneal cavities of immune A2G mice up to the 4th day after challenge. We found it difficult to explain why the number of tumor cells did not become even further reduced in passively immunized A2G mice during the observation period of 80 hours. These animals should eventually have eliminated all tumor cells since similarly protected controls did survive the challenge dose. Perhaps the interaction of A2G anti-EA antibody and tumor cells released immunogenic materials which later resulted in a superimposed active immunization. It is also possible that the elimination of tumor cells by host cells took longer than 80 hours.

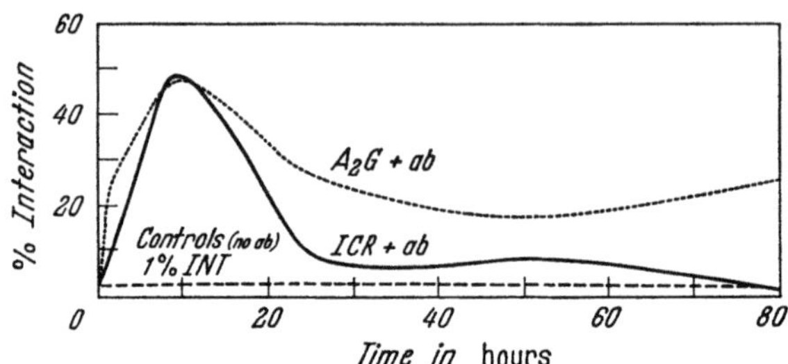

Fig. 15c. Aggregation of host cells around tumor cells in passively immunized and control A2G and ICR mice. These studies were performed on the peritoneal cell populations of the tumor bearing animals examined in Figs. 15a and 15b, and at the same time intervals (1, 9, 23, 44 and 80 hours). — Smears from the peritoneal exudates of individual mice were fixed and stained with Giemsa stain. For each exudate differential counts were made on 128 low power fields. Free tumor cells and tumor cells with one or more host cells adhering to their surface were counted. The % interaction was expressed:

$$\frac{\text{No. of tumor cells with one or more attached host cells}}{\text{total No. of tumor cells counted}} \times 100$$

When antibody was omitted from the system, the % interaction remained below 1% for the entire observation period in both A2G and ICR mice (broken line)

The predominant host cells during the first 24—48 hours of i. p. tumor residence in the presence of immune serum were polymorphonuclear leukocytes. An invasion by macrophages occurred somewhat later (72 hours). We have observed neither the occurrence of "giant cells" nor of phagocytosis of tumor cells during this experiment. This does not mean, however, that such phenomena are unimportant in postoncolytic immunity. We shall present direct evidence in a later section that phagocytosis of both tumor debris and virus particles did occur following viral oncolysis (p. 57).

Figure 15b shows the behavior of the A2G anti-EA agglutinin in tumor-bearing and tumor-free A2G and ICR mice. The tumor-bearing mice were the same mice used for Figure 15a. Each mouse received 3000 "agglutinating units" of antibody at 0 hour. It is apparent that a ten-fold dilution of the agglutinin occurred *in vivo*. We chose to follow the agglutinin rather than the anti-ε precipitin for two reasons. First, we had shown that there was a positive correlation between the agglutinin titer of A2G immune sera and its protective capacity *in vivo* (see p. 35), but we lacked similar evidence for the anti-ε precipitin. Second, our best A2G anti-ε serum had a precipitin titer of only 1:10. Considering the *in vivo* dilution factor to be encountered our choice was obvious.

Circulating agglutinin levels of almost identical magnitude were reached within 1 hour in all mice tested. The clearance of the agglutinin proceeded at a rather sluggish rate in syngeneic A2G mice without the tumor. The half life of the antibody in such mice was certainly greater than 3 days. This clearance rate is similar to that observed in other strains of mice (TEE et al., 1965; SPIEGELBERG and WEIGLE, 1965). In allogeneic, non-protectable ICR mice without tumors 50% of the antibody had been cleared from the circulation within 17 hours and at 40 hours the antibody could no longer be detected. In A2G mice bearing the tumor agglutinin levels remained constant for the first 24 hours. The agglutinin titer proceeded to drop for the next 20 hours but then remained stable at levels 2 to 4-fold below the initial value. In ICR tumor-bearing mice with immune serum, however, the picture was quite different. The agglutinin levels remained constant for only the first 10 hours after which they dropped steadily until they could no longer be detected at 80 hours.

Although ICR mice cleared A2G agglutinating antibody at an astonishing rate, we had no idea if this represented clearance of specific antibody or if this was the manner in which such mice clear A2G γ-globulin in general. The fate of A2G specific antibody directed against non-cellular antigens must be followed to decide this issue. Such experiments are currently in progress in our laboratories.

We did know, however, that ICR mice shared the ε-alloantigen with the tumor cells used. It became tempting then to imagine that perhaps the unusually rapid clearance of the agglutinin in ICR mice was due to its absorption *in vivo* by an antigen common to some normal ICR tissues and the tumor cells. This would explain why ICR mice and certain other strains could not be protected passively by A2G anti-EA immune serum, and why the initial inhibition of the tumor's growth rate was not maintained in ICR mice (Fig. 15a). The difference in antibody clearance kinetics between tumor-bearing and tumor-free ICR mice could be explained by imagining that some of the agglutinin was rapidly bound onto tumor cells. During destruction of tumor cells by host defense mechanisms part of the tumor-bound antibody might be liberated to again compete for the host's antigen and its counterpart on tumor cells. In this way a gradual disappearance of the agglutinin might be explained. If similar events also took place in tumor-bearing A2G mice, the antibody thus set free would be available for "full-time duty" as an anti-tumor agent since it should not be absorbed by any common antigen in A2G tissues.

Figure 15c presents a record of the tumor cell-host cell interplay observed during the course of the experiment in both ICR and A2G mice. By the 15th hour after challenge approximately 50 % of the tumor cells in both mouse strains were contacted on their surface by peritoneal host cells. In tumor-bearing mice not treated with A2G anti-EA antibody such interactions occurred in fewer than 1 % of tumor cells.

Since peritoneal cells of both mouse strains were equally competent in "contacting" tumor cells during the first 15 hours of the experiment, some other explanation for the non-protectability of ICR mice must be sought. A decrease in the intensity of interaction was observed in both strains after the 15th hour. However, this decline leveled off in A2G mice so that by the 80th hour, 25 % of the tumor cells were still being acted upon by A2G peritoneal cells. On the other hand, the interaction rapidly declined to levels below 10 % in ICR mice and became negligible by 80 hours. These interactions curves paralleled the behavior of the agglutinin described in Figure 15b.

The following tentative picture of passive protection by postoncolytic antibody emerges. In A2G mice passively treated with A2G anti-EA serum, agglutinin levels high enough to mediate the interplay between host cells and tumor cells are maintained for a considerable length of time. In ICR mice, the rapid clearance of agglutinin from the circulation interrupts the "immune" reactions between host cells and tumor cells, thereby preventing successful passive protection of the host. The mechanism of agglutinin clearance may indeed be absorption *in vivo* by an antigen shared by tumor and host. If this is so then we might predict that only those strains which are passively protectable can be actively immunized against the tumor. This of course assumes that all strains are equally capable of synthesizing the antibody molecule when stimulated with the immunogen. We shall consider this point more closely later in our discussion of reovirus oncolysis (p. 62).

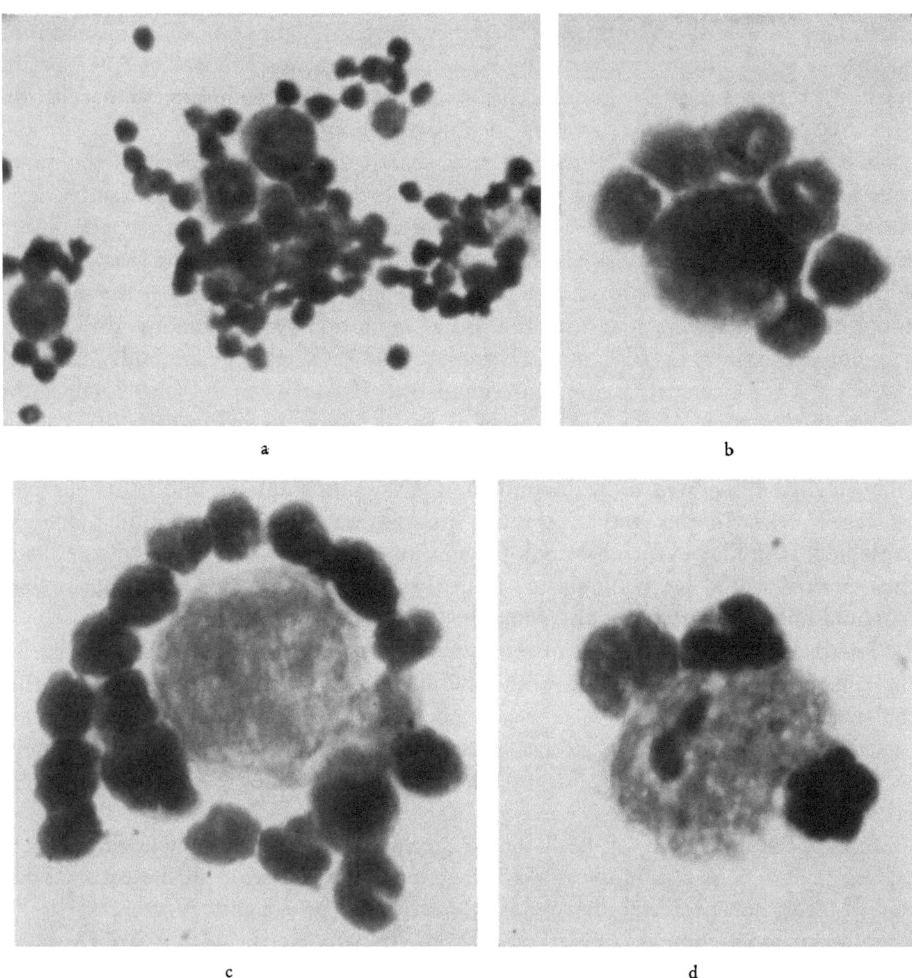

Fig. 16. *In vivo* interaction of A2G and ICR peritoneal cells (mainly polymorphonuclear leucocytes) with Ehrlich ascites tumor cells in the presence of A2G anti-EA antiserum. — a) Attachment of A2G peritoneal cells onto Ehrlich tumor cells 13 hours after intraperitoneal injection of the tumor cells and A2G anti-tumor antiserum. 600× (2/3). — b) Same experiment as Fig. 16a, but performed in an ICR mouse. 1,800× (2/3). — c) and d) Further example of A2G peritoneal cells clustering around Ehrlich tumor cells. 1,800× (2/3)

Figure 16 shows some of the interactions observed between A2G and ICR peritoneal cells and Ehrlich tumor cells 13 hours after challenge of passively immunized animals. Polymorphonuclear leukocytes predominated at this early hour. It was difficult to decide if localized breakdown of the cytoplasmic membrane between host and tumor cells occurred here as it did in the case of the L1210 ascites system (JOURNEY and AMOS, 1962). Electron microscopic analysis of such interactions should be enlightening on this point.

f) Immunogenicity of Viral Oncolysates

We have seen in the previous sections that mice which had survived oncolysis became solidly immune to tumor challenge. In order to learn more about the nature and the state of the antigens present in viral oncolysates, we tried as it were to divide the experiment among different animals. Thus the acute phase of oncolysis, the interaction between tumor cells and virus, would take place in a first set of animals. The product of virus-tumor interaction (the viral oncolysate) would then be inoculated into a second set of animals in an attempt to induce immunity. The subdivision into an early phase of oncolysis and a later phase of developing immunity was to some extent arbitrary. We usually let the virus act upon tumor cells for 48 to 72 hours, collected the solidified masses of tumor debris, homogenized them and used this as a vaccine to immunize A2G mice. It is, of course, impossible to state categorically that important steps of the immune reaction had not already begun during the oncolytic phase. The experiments would be much more elegant if the first phase had been done entirely *in vitro*. We have not yet embarked upon such experiments mainly for quantitative reasons. It is difficult to maintain tumor cell population densities of more than 10^6 cells per ml for any length of time in vitro. By contrast, tumor ascites easily accomodates 10^8 cells per ml. We therefore expected more clear cut results from experiments using *in vivo* oncolysis. It should be noted, however, that Krebs-2 ascites tumor cells treated *in vitro* with influenza virus and then injected into mice have been shown to be immunogenic, although the nature of the antigens involved remains unknown (EATON et al., 1965). To our knowledge experiments involving the immunogenicity of viral oncolysates produced *in vivo* have not been previously reported. The series of investigations which we have started is at this writing far from being complete. The results are sufficiently suggestive, however, to warrant their inclusion here (KLEIN and LINDENMANN, unpublished).

WSA oncolysates of Ehrlich cells were produced by inoculating A2G or ICR mice bearing 8 day ascites tumors i. p. with 50 to 100 EID_{50}'s of the virus. 48 to 72 hours later the peritoneal contents of these mice were harvested. The oncolysate was then homogenized with a teflon-glass apparatus in order to break open residual tumor cells. After freezing and thawing once, and centrifuging at 15 000 g for 15', the supernatant fluid was frozen at —70 °C for future use. Oncolysates thus prepared contained approximately 2×10^8 Ehrlich cell equivalents per milliliter, had hemagglutination titers of 1:200 to 1:2500 and infectivity titers between 10^8 and 10^9 EID_{50} per ml.

A2G mice were immunized with these oncolysates via the intraperitoneal route according to several schedules. They were challenged 10 to 28 days after oncolysate injection with various numbers of viable Ehrlich tumor cells and followed for 30 days to see if they would develop tumors. Repeated challenges were given at 30 days' intervals. Table 12 gives the results of a typical immunization experiment using two different oncolysate preparations.

A single injection of 0.5 ml of oncolysate III (8×10^7 EA cell equivalents) immunized most A2G mice against 1000 EA cells (100 LD_{50}'s), but failed to induce immunity against challenge with 100 000 tumor cells (10 000 LD_{50}'s). Four injections of oncolysate III spaced at weekly intervals enabled the majority of mice to resist challenge with both 1000 and 100 000 tumor cell doses. Results of oncolysate II are included mainly to demonstrate that resistance to challenge with 10^6 tumor cells could be induced provided multiple challenges with lower doses had first been given.

Table 12. *Active Immunization of A2G Mice against Ehrlich Ascites Tumor with Viral Oncolysates*

Type of immunization[a]	1st chall. 10^3 cells	10^5 cells	2nd chall. 10^5 cells	3rd chall. 10^6 cells
WSA EA oncolysate II (HA titer 1:200)				
0.3 ml i.p. 4×	10/10 [b]	n. d. [c]	9/10	7/9
WSA EA oncolysate III (HA titer 1:1600)				
0.4 ml i.p. 1×	9/10	0/10 [d]	8/9	n. d.
WSA EA oncolysate III (HA titer 1:1600)				
0.4 ml i.p. 4×	9/10	9/9 [e]	12/16	n. d.
None (control)	0/10	0/10	0/10	n. d.

[a] EA tumor was grown in ICR mice and infected with WSA virus. The oncolytic tumor was harvested after 48 hours and used as a vaccine as described in the text.

[b] No. of mice protected / No. of mice in each group.

[c] n. d. = not done.

[d] 5 died of subcutaneous tumor and not ascites.

[e] 2 died of subcutaneous tumors 79 days after challenge.

Table 13. *Control Experiments for Viral Oncolysate Immunizations*

Description of experiment	Result
A. Immunization with egg grown WSA virus (HA titer 1:80) 0.5 ml i.p. 4×; challenge with 1000 EA cells i.p.	0/18 [a]
B. 10^4 EA cells + WSA virus on day 0; challenge on day 28 with 1000 EA cells i.p.	0/7 [a]
C. 10^6 EA cells + WSA virus on day 0	All 7 mice dead of ascites by day 28 (before intended challenge)
D. 2.5×10^6 EA cells + WSA virus on day 0; challenge survivors on day 28 with 20,000 EA cells i.p.	1/5 dead by day 28 (before challenge) 4/5 resist challenge
E. 1.0 ml of viral oncolysate III i.p. to mice actively immunized against WSA virus	9/10 survive 90 days with no sign of tumor. 1/10 dead of ascites by day 33 (no challenge)
F. 0.4 ml of viral oncolysate III + 1000 EA cells i.p. to mice pre-immunized against WSA virus	All 5 mice dead of ascites by day 28 (no challenge)

[a] No. of mice protected / No. of mice in each group (all mice were A2G).

In all cases circulating anti-EA agglutinin could be detected 9 days after a single oncolysate injection. Anti-ε was not detectable under the same conditions. We have observed generally that those oncolysates with the highest virus titers were the best immunogenic preparations. Thus an oncolysate with an HA titer of 1:2500 could induce resistance to 1000 LD_{50}'s of tumor in 100 % of mice treated with 0.5 ml of this preparation given once intraperitoneally. A similar preparation with an HA titer of 1:200 induced resistance in only 25 % of such animals under the same conditions.

At this point several control experiments should be considered. For example, when 10^8 physically lysed cell equivalents or 1000 HA units of egg-grown WSA were injected repeatedly i. p. into A2G mice, tumor immunity failed to develop. Table 13 lists additional types of control experiments we have carried out.

Immunization with egg-grown WSA failed to induce tumor immunity (A). It is clear from experiment E that oncolysate III contained few viable tumor cells. We have already stated that viral oncolysis could not occur in the presence of circulating antiviral antibody (LINDENMANN, 1963). Hence any viable tumor cells in a viral oncolysate should be free to grow in mice actively immunized against the virus.

Experiment B points out that viral oncolysis of 10^4 EA cells was insufficient to effect immunization against the tumor. Even 10^6 EA cells apparently lead to the release of only a sub-threshold dose of immunogen (experiment C). Whereas the virus seemed able to cope with 10^4 EA cells (experiment B), it was unable to destroy a sufficiently large proportion of 10^6 cells; in fact, all animals succumbed before we had a chance to challenge them (experiment C). Paradoxically, when even more tumor cells were added (2.5×10^6, experiment D), only one mouse died before challenge, and the four survivors resisted challenge with 2×10^4 tumor cells. 2.5×10^6 tumor cells is probably close to the minimum number which must be lysed by virus to induce antitumor immunity. These observations also explain why oncolysis performed a few days after tumor implantation resulted in more "cures" than earlier treatment.

Finally, experiment F tested the possibility that the viral oncolysate itself contained anti-EA immune globulin and that what we were observing was passive protection rather than active immunization. Since an "immunogenic dose" of the oncolysate failed to protect WSA-immune A2G mice against as few as 1000 cells given concurrently, we can safely assume that immune antitumor globulin was absent from such a preparation. This result also points out that active immunization must be achieved some time before the mouse is given even a small challenge dose of tumor cells. Apparently even these small tumor doses can "outrace" the developing immunity and kill the host.

As we shall demonstrate, there is a remarkable difference in the resistance induced in A2G mice by mechanical and viral lysates of equivalent numbers of tumor cells. For example, mice receiving the equivalent of 10^8 cells in the form of a viral oncolysate could resist a primary challenge with up to 10 000 tumor cells (1000 LD$_{50}$). The same number of cell equivalents given in the form of a physical lysate of cells (either untreated or CHCl$_3$-extracted) failed to induce immunity to even 1000 cells by several routes thus far explored (KLEIN, 1965).

We have recently completed an interesting experiment which we present in Table 14. This was designed to test whether or not DEAE cellulose chromatography could be used to separate the immunogen from either the virus particle or the ε-alloantigen in a WSA oncolysate of the Ehrlich tumor. An oncolysate with an HA titer of 1:2500 was applied to a column of DEAE cellulose and then eluted stepwise with phosphate buffers containing increasing concentrations of NaCl.

3 ml fractions were collected and these were assayed for virus infectivity, hemagglutinin titer, the ε-alloantigen and for ability to induce tumor immunity in A2G

mice. Challenge doses of 1000 EA cells (100 LD$_{50}$'s) were used in all cases to assess resistance to tumor growth. The elution behavior of WSA on DEAE cellulose as observed here was similar to that of many myxoviruses (F. Sokol, personal com-

Table 14. *Fractionation of a WSA EA Oncolysate by Chromatography on DEAE Cellulose*

Fract. No.	Molar. in NaCl	Hemaggl. titer	Infectivity [a]	ε-antigen detectable [b]	Anti-tumor immunogenic activity [c]
9	0.01	1:16	—	+	—
28	0.03	1:8	—	+	—
44	0.05	1:4	—	—	—
61	0.07	1:4	—	—	—
78	0.10	1:8	+	—	—
98	0.15	1:8	+	—	—
112	0.20	1:16	+	—	—
130	0.30	1:32	+	—	+
155	0.50	1:16	+	—	+
167	1.00	1:8	+	—	—

[a] Measured by intracerebral inoculation of 0.03 ml of undiluted peak fraction into ICR mice. Inoculum was first dialysed against 0.15 M NaCl. + means that animals died of WSA infection.

[b] Measured by gel diffusion assay of 10✕ concentrated peak fraction against A2G anti-ε antibody.

[c] Measured by ability of injected peak fraction to prime A2G mice to make anti-EA agglutinating antibody upon challenge with 1000 live EA tumor cells and to resist such challenge.

munication). Virus-specific hemagglutinin was eluted at molarities 0.10 to 1.00. The non-specific hemagglutinin in the first 4 fractions was probably similar to that previously described as a component of normal A2G serum (LINDENMANN et al., 1963). The ε-alloantigen was eluted with 0.01 M and 0.03 M NaCl concentrations as previously discussed (see section b). None of the fractions induced detectable pre-challenge levels of agglutinating or anti-ε antibodies. Mice "primed" with fractions 130 and 157 had detectable levels of anti-EA agglutinin by the 12th day after tumor challenge. Mice in these two groups were the only ones to survive the challenge dose of 1000 tumor cells. All mice in other groups succumbed to the tumor within the usual length of time. There was no evidence of either agglutinin formation or delayed tumor deaths in mice receiving ε-containing fractions.

It is difficult to use this experiment for a final decision on the role of the ε-alloantigen in the induction of tumor immunity. The fact seems clear that ε-rich fractions were unable to induce agglutinin formation or tumor immunity under the conditions of the experiment. It may yet be that ε was incorporated into the envelopes of immunogenic virus particles in active fractions 130 and 155 and that it was in this form that it induced agglutinin formation and tumor immunity. Moreover, the experiment failed to decide whether the factor which immunized the mice against the tumor was independent of or integrated into the WSA virus particle. We present this experiment only to illustrate one of the approaches we have taken with this problem and to indicate the many factors which must be considered before final judgment is made on the role of any one component in postoncolytic immunity.

g) Tumor Immunity Following Reovirus Oncolysis

Up to this point we have reported on experiments done with WSA virus as the oncolytic agent and A2G mice as hosts. The use of A2G mice was mandatory since they belonged to the only known influenza virus resistant strain (LINDENMANN and KLEIN, 1966). When we learned of the oncolytic capacities of a reovirus, we thought that it might provide an independent check on some of the more puzzling features that had emerged from our previous work. In particular, we wanted to know if there would be any correlation between the ability of certain strains to be protected passively and their ability to be immunized actively against the same tumor. Furthermore, we felt it important to test the effectiveness of an entirely different virus in inducing postoncolytic immunity in order to see if differences in virus morphology and physiology would influence the final outcome.

In 1960, BENNETTE had reported the isolation of an oncolytic agent which was non-pathogenic for mice. One of the most interesting properties of this agent was its ability to grow in and destroy a wide variety of different tumors. The agent has been identified as a reovirus type 3 (Bennette, personal communication) as has the oncolytic agent isolated by NELSON and TARNOVSKI (1960), (HARTLEY et al., 1961). We have been able to confirm this finding with the generous help of Dr. L. Rosen. Findings of postoncolytic immunity using this virus have not been reported previously.

Experiments with this virus were carried out using the Sa 180 tumor growing in various strains of mice (KLEIN, in press). Most often, experiments designed to measure the nature of postoncolytic immunity were carried out in A2G or A/Jax

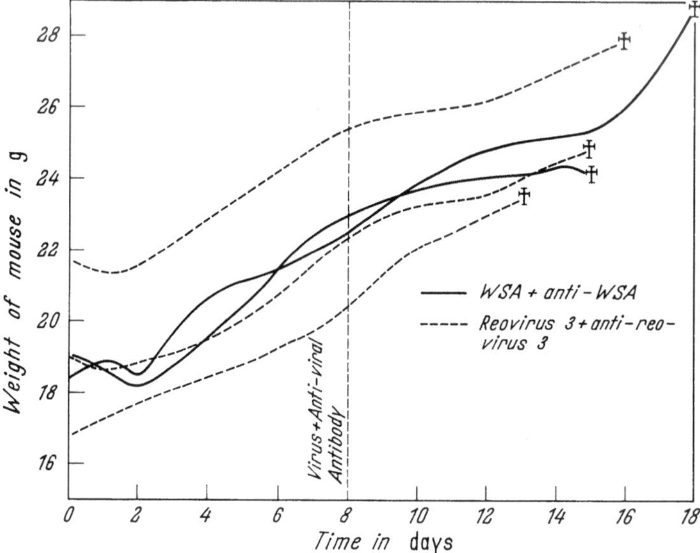

Fig. 17. Weight curves of individual A/Jax mice bearing Sarcoma 180 ascites tumors and treated either with WSA virus + mouse anti-WSA serum (solid lines) or with reovirus type 3 + mouse anti-reo 3 serum (broken lines). All mice had received inoculations of 10^6 viable tumor cells on day 0. Crosses mark the day of death. The anti-WSA serum used was of ICR origin, had an HI titer of 1 : 640 and was used against 100 ID_{50} (see legend to Fig. 18) of WSA. The anti-reovirus serum was of A/Jax origin, had an HI titer of 1 : 5000 and was used against 1000 TID_{50} (see legend to Fig. 18) of reovirus type 3. The sera did not cross-react. Note absence of oncolysis. Compare with Fig. 18 for effect of the viruses when no antiserum was added

mice. The LD$_{50}$ of the Sa 180 tumor in A/Jax mice was similar to that reported for A2G mice. Thus challenge doses of 1000 tumor cells uniformly killed 100 % of mice from either strain. Figure 17 shows that both the reovirus and the WSA virus were unable to effect oncolysis when given to tumor-bearing mice along with their corresponding anti-viral antibody.

Cross-neutralization experiments revealed that these antisera were indeed specific: Anti-reovirus type 3 antiserum was unable to neutralize the oncolytic or hemagglutinating activities of WSA virus and vice versa. Figure 18 shows that tumor-bearing A/Jax mice unable to survive oncolysis by neuropathogenic WSA could be "cured" of their tumors by the non-pathogenic reovirus.

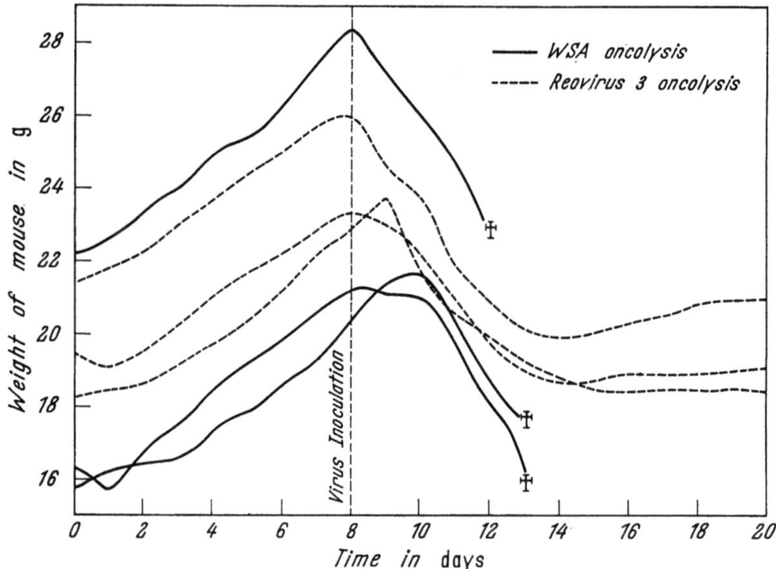

Fig. 18. Weight curves of individual A/Jax mice bearing Sarcoma 180 ascites tumors and treated either with WSA virus (solid lines) or with reovirus type 3 (broken lines). All mice had received inoculations of 10^6 viable tumor cells on day 0. Mice treated with WSA virus received 100 ID$_{50}$ as measured by intracerebral titrations in ICR mice. Mice treated with reovirus type 3 received 1000 TID$_{50}$ (50% tumor infectious dose) as measured by intraperitoneal titration in tumor-bearing ICR mice. Crosses mark the day of death. Note oncolysis as evidenced by rapid weight loss. A/Jax mice, which are fully susceptible to WSA virus, died during the acute phase of oncolysis

Although oncolysis by reovirus was initiated here on the 8th day, the highest proportion of "cures" was achieved by treating mice on the 4th day after tumor inoculation. As has been described for WSA oncolysis a certain proportion of mice surviving reovirus oncolysis developed subcutaneous tumors along the tumor inoculation needle track and eventually succumbed to these growths. A satisfactory explanation of this perplexing phenomenon has not yet been found.

The development of the reovirus in Ehrlich tumor cells was followed with the electron microscope. We are indebted to Dr. J. W. Shands for his efforts in preparing the following electron micrographs. Oncolysates were harvested at various times following reovirus inoculation of tumor-bearing mice. They were fixed in glutaraldehyde and post-fixed with osmium tetroxide. After staining with uranyl acetate and lead citrate, they were embedded in Epon for sectioning. Figure 19 shows the development of the virus within vesicles in the cytoplasm of the tumor cell.

Early stages in the degeneration of the tumor are suggested by Figure 20. Figure 21 presents the picture of a typical reovirus oncolysate 88 hours after virus inoculation.

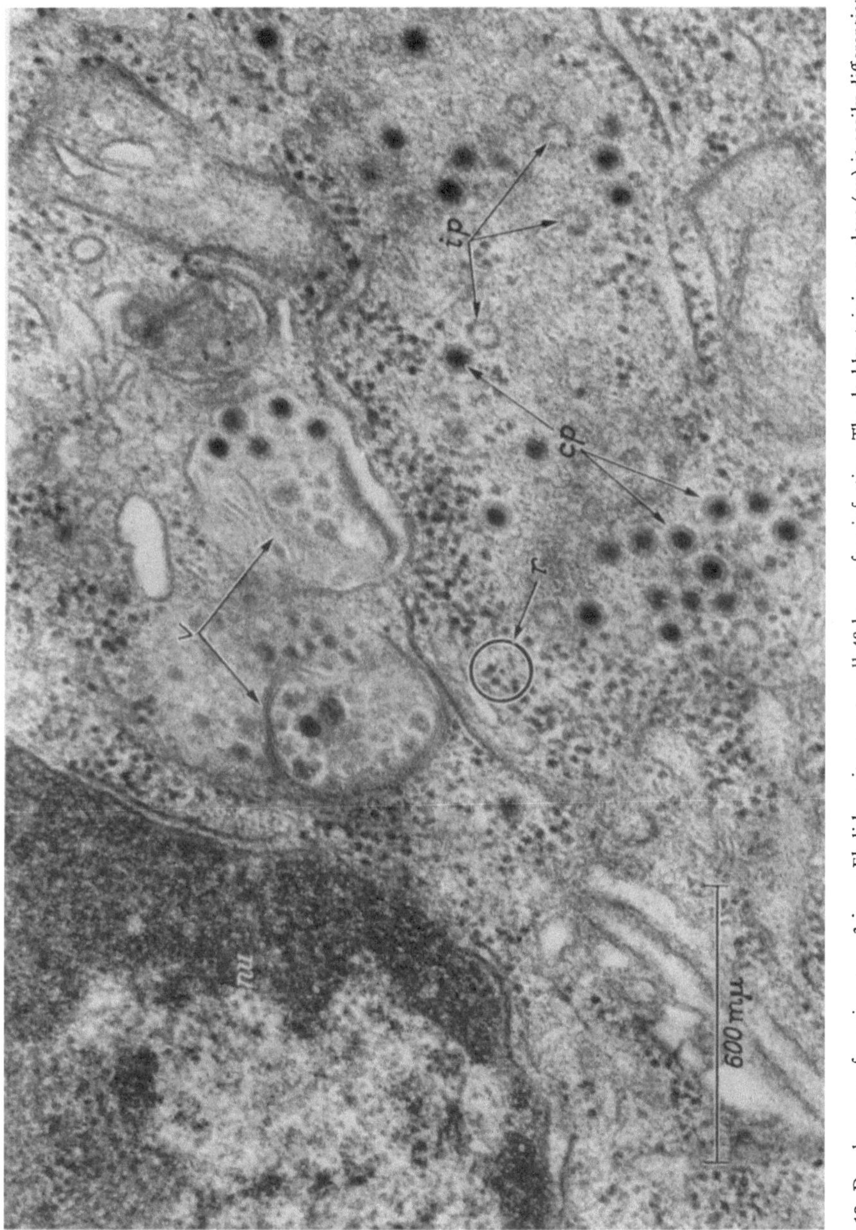

Fig. 19. Development of reovirus type 3 in an Ehrlich ascites tumor cell 48 hours after infection. The darkly staining nucleus (nu) is easily differentiated from the cytoplasm which contains numerous ribosomes (r). Both complete (cp) and incomplete (ip) virus particles are visible within the cytoplasm. The development and maturation of the virus appear to take place within vesicles (v) or cavities situated near the nucleus and bound by multiple membranes. The mechanism of virus release from these structures is not clear

Figure 22 provides our first direct evidence that phagocytosis of both virus particles and tumor debris occurred following virus oncolysis.

A2G and A/Jax mice surviving reovirus oncolysis of Sa 180 proved to be resistant to challenge with 10^6 tumor cells (100 000 LD$_{50}$'s) given 60 days after oncolysis. Suitable control experiments have been carried out to insure that the observed immunity was not due to residual reovirus within postoncolytic survivors.

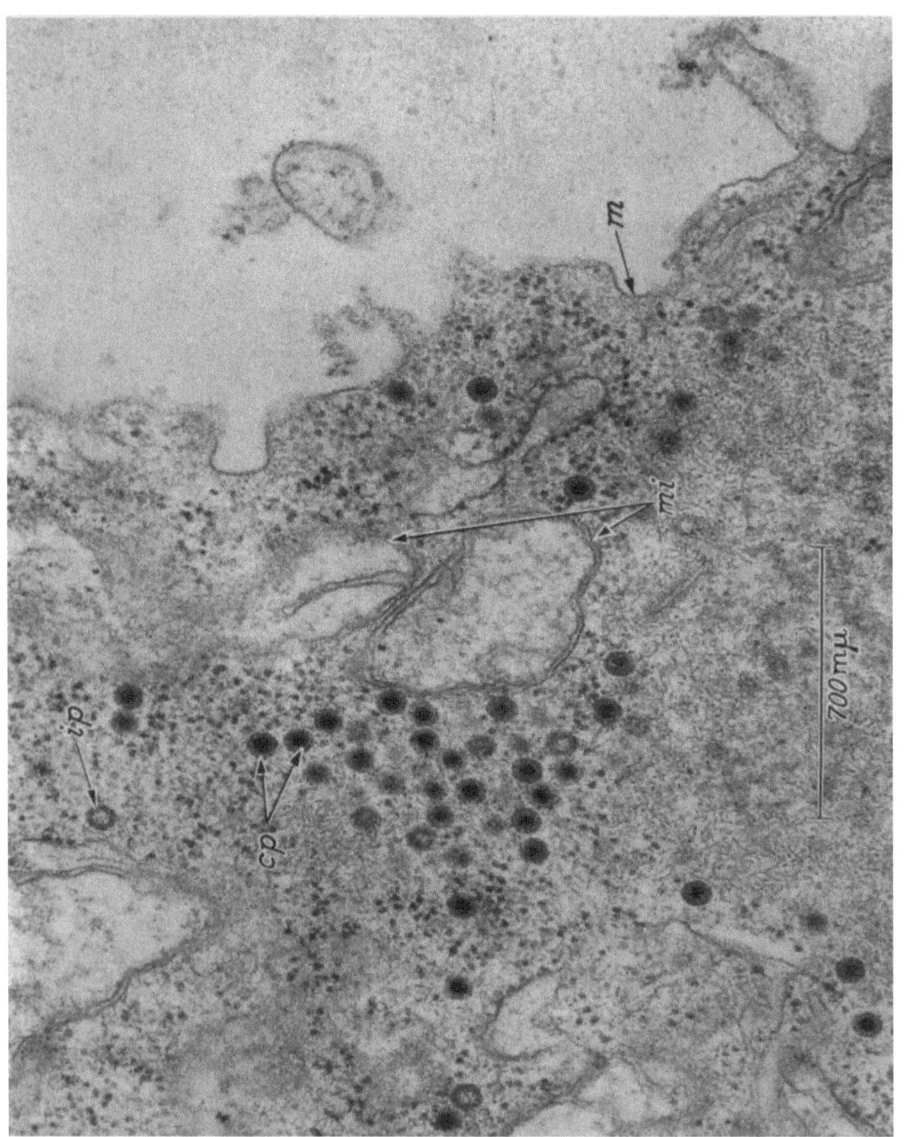

Fig. 20. Reovirus particles, both complete (cp) and incomplete (ip), in Ehrlich ascites tumor cell 40 hours after infection. Breaks in the cell membrane (m) cannot be attributed to the virus. Degenerating mitochondria (mi) are visible within the cytoplasm

Mice surviving reovirus oncolysis of Sa 180 proved to be resistant to challenge with EA tumor. A tumor agglutinin and an anti-ε precipitating antibody were detectable in postoncolytic immune sera. The sera of such mice were able to protect passively mice of strain A or A2G against challenge with EA. Mice of strain ICR, on the other hand, proved to be non-protectable with the same sera. The Krebs-2 tumor was not tested in this system.

An immune ascitic fluid pool was obtained from several A/Jax mice which had survived repeated challenge with both Sa 180 and EA. This fluid had a tumor

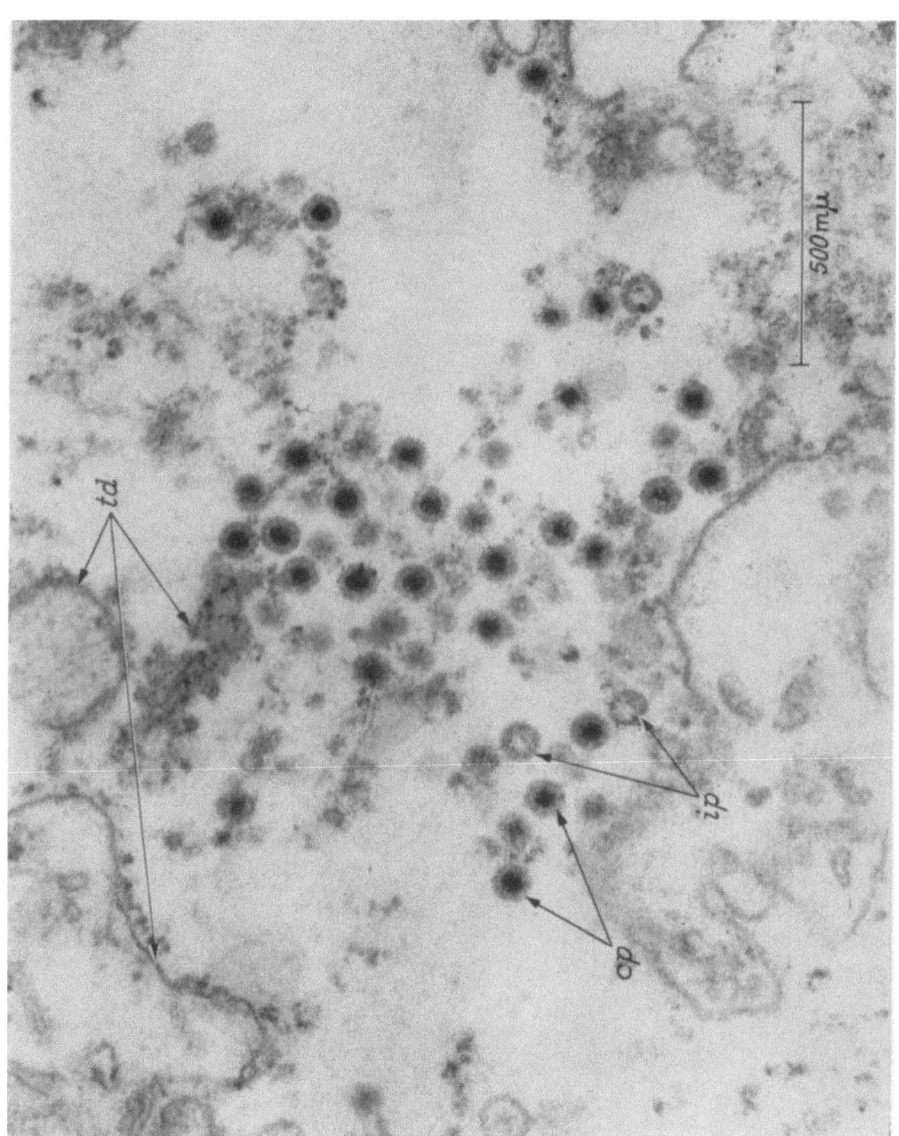

Fig. 21. Reovirus oncolysate produced by in vitro destruction of Ehrlich ascites tumor cells, 72 hours after infection. Visible are both complete (cp) and incomplete (ip) particles of reovirus type 3. Tumor debris (td) is scattered throughout and seems to consist of cytoplasmic fragments, disintegrated cell organelles and pieces of membranes

agglutination titer of 1:1000, but no detectable anti-ε precipitin. The γ globulin fraction was obtained by a combination of salt fractionation and DEAE cellulose chromatography. A single peak was obtained following gel-filtration chromatography of the globulin in Sephadex G-200. Figure 23 gives the result of this experiment.

Fractions no. 33—41 from the column were pooled, concentrated to 2 mg/ml, and analyzed by immunoelectrophoresis against two rabbit antisera to whole A2G serum and one goat anti-mouse globulin serum. Figure 24 shows that at a concen-

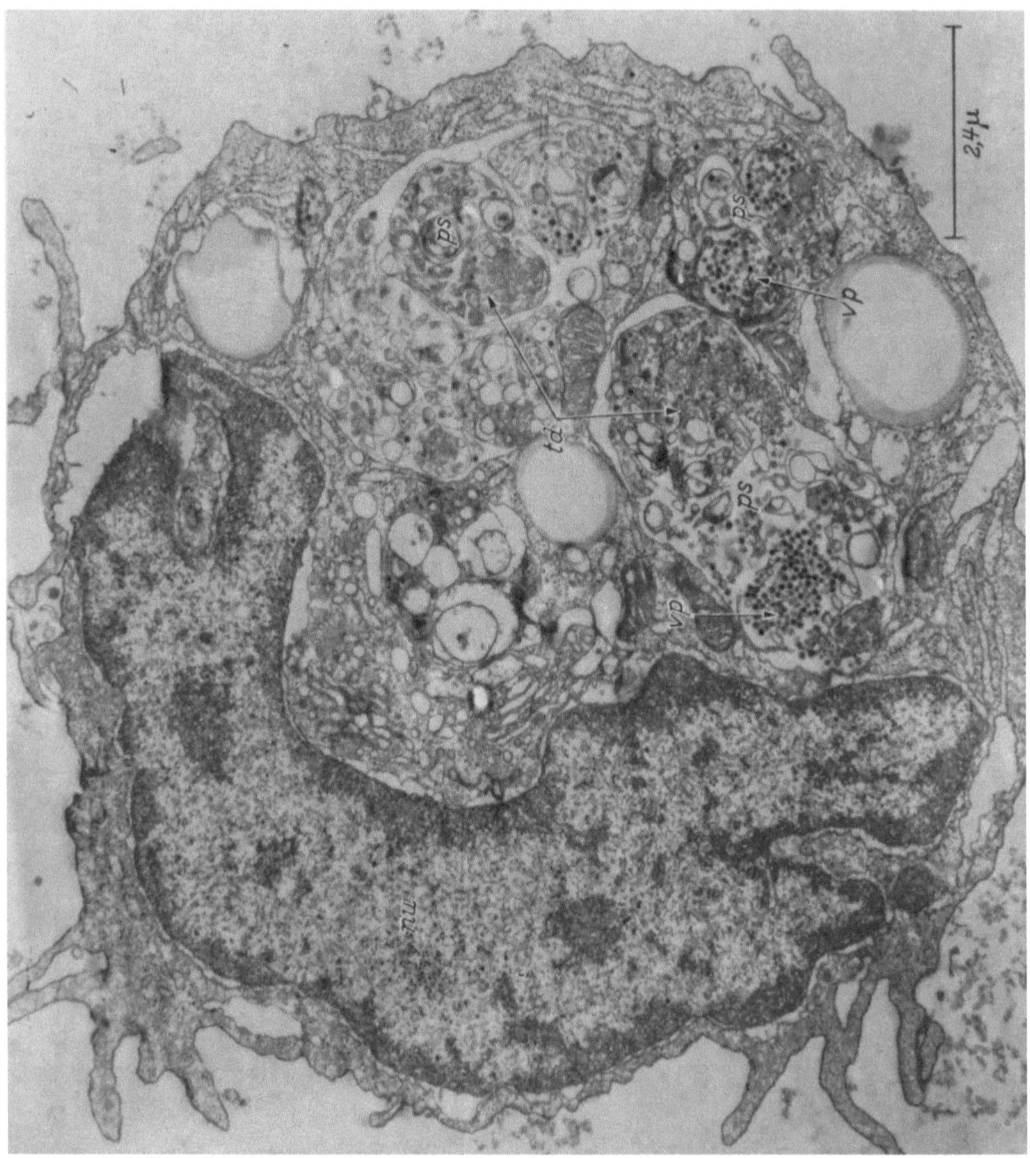

Fig. 22. Phagocytosis of a reovirus oncolysate of Ehrlich ascites tumor by an A/Jax macrophage *in vivo*, 88 hours after infection. The nucleus

tration of 0.25 mg/ml the pool contained a single component with the mobility of γ G mouse immunoglobulin. However, at a concentration of 2 mg/ml (not shown) an additional "spur" was detected originating from the major band seen in this figure.

These two components appeared to correspond to the $7S\gamma_1$ and $7S\gamma_2$ globulins of the mouse as described by FAHEY et al. (1964).

Ultracentrifugal analysis of the pool at a concentration of 2 mg/ml revealed the presence of a single component with a sedimentation coefficient of 7.1 S (Figure 25).

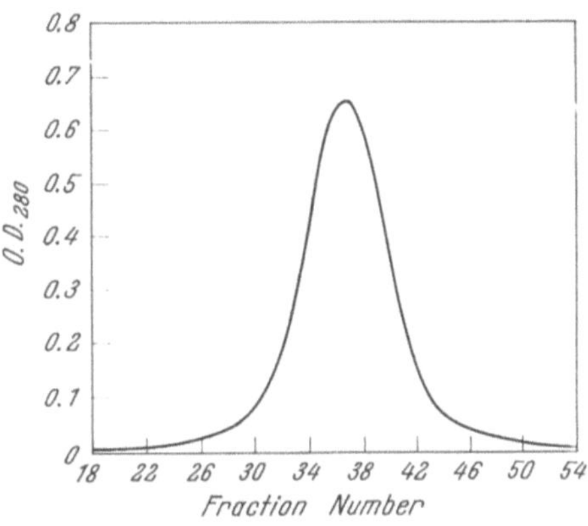

Fig. 23. Fractionation of A/Jax anti-Sa 180 gamma-globulin on a column of Sephadex G-200. 25.5 mg of gamma-globulin were applied to a column of 2.5×90 cm in a volume of 5.8 ml. This sample had been prepared by DEAE cellulose chromatography of a 0.37 saturated $(NH_4)_2SO_4$ precipitate of an A/Jax postreovirus oncolysis hyperimmune ascites pool. The Sephadex G-200 column and the sample were equilibrated in 0.1 M phosphate buffer pH 6.8. Fractions of 5 ml were collected. Fractions No. 33—41 were pooled and concentrated to 2 mg of gamma-globulin per ml. The molecular homogeneity of the pool was assessed by immunoelectrophoresis (see Fig. 24) and by ultracentrifugation (see Fig. 25). The ability of the pool to agglutinite Sarcoma 180 tumor cells *in vitro* and to protect passively A/Jax mice against challenge with viable tumor cells was also tested (see text)

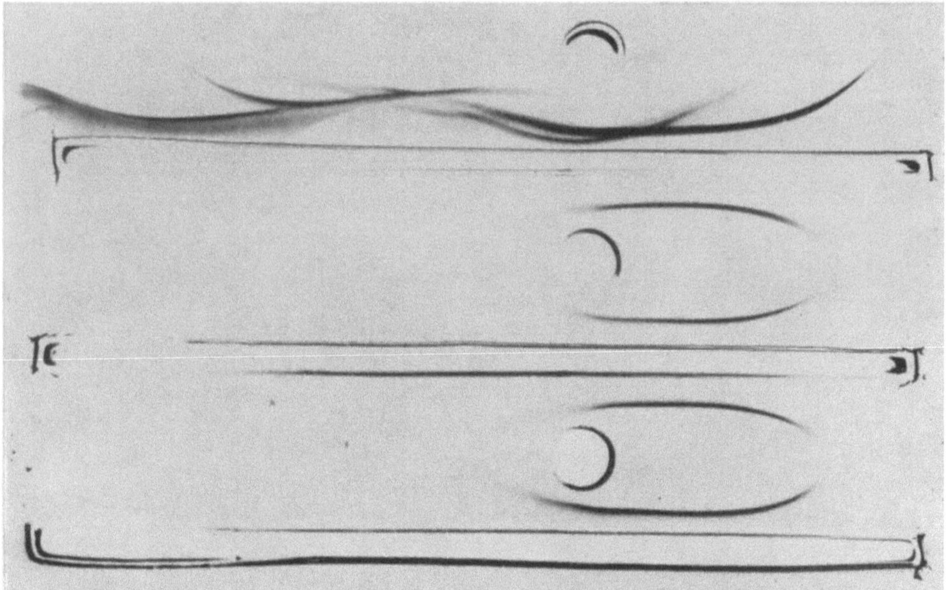

Fig. 24. Immunoelectrophoresis or normal A2G whole serum and chromatographically pure A/Jax anti-Sa 180 gamma-globulin (see Figs. 23 and 25). Supporting medium was Ionagar gel in Veronal buffer pH 8.6. Anode to the left, 15 mA 2 hrs. The reaction was developed for 48 hours before being photographed. — Upper well: A2G whole serum. Center and lower well: A/Jax anti-Sa 180 gamma-globulin. Upper and lower trough: Rabbit antiserum against whole mouse serum. Center trough: Goat antiserum against mouse gamma-globulin

With this preparation, which had a tumor agglutination titer of 1:50 at 1 mg/ml, we have thus far been able to protect A/Jax mice against 10 000 Sa 180 cells with as little as $50\mu g$ of γ-globulin per mouse.

Tumor immunity following reovirus oncolysis of nonspecific tumors was thus similar to that following WSA oncolysis. Both seemed to be mediated by humoral factors identifiable as 7 S immunoglobulins. A tumor agglutinin was regularly found in the postoncolytic serum of both systems, and an anti-ε precipitin was frequently present. The same mouse strains were passively protectable or proved refractory to

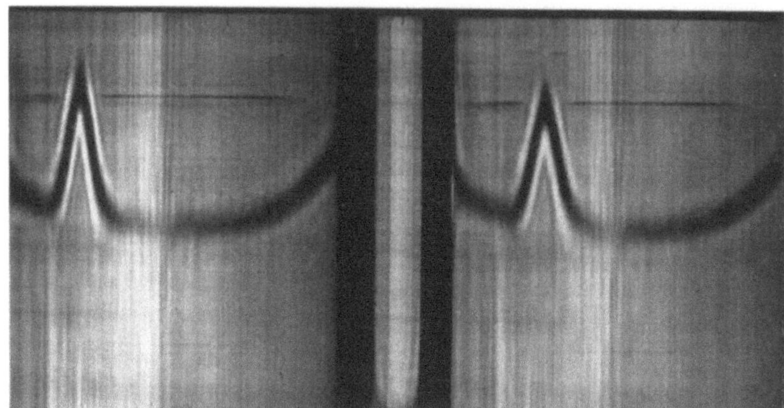

Fig. 25. Schlieren patterns obtained from sedimentation velocity experiments with A/Jax anti-Sa 180 gamma-globulin (see Figs. 23 and 24). Speed 56,100 rpm, temperature 20.0° C. Bar angle 35°. Concentration 2.0 mg of gamma-globulin per ml in 0.1 M phosphate buffer pH 6.8. The photo on the left was taken 32 minutes after reaching set speed, the photo on the right 8 minutes later. The $S_{20,\,w}$ value of the peak is 7.1 S

passive protection in either case. We have no definite proof, however, that the protective antibodies induced by the two viruses were directed against the same antigenic target on the tumor cell.

Table 15. *Ability of Various Inbred Strains of Mice to Respond with Protective Antibody Production Following Reovirus Oncolysis of Sarcoma 180*

Mouse strain	Presence of ε-alloantigen	Anti-Reovirus response[a]	Anti-Sa 180 response[b]
A2G/Dub	—	+	+
A/Jax	—	+	+
C3H/HeJ	—	+	+
RF/J	—	+	—
(RF×A2G)F1	--	+	—
DBA/2J	+	+	—
ICR/Dub [b]	+	+	—

[a] As measured by increase in hemagglutination-inhibition titers.

[b] As measured *in vitro* by slide agglutination of tumor cells and *in vivo* by passive protection of A/Jax mice.

[c] Non-inbred.

Because of the non-pathogenicity of the reovirus we have been able to study the development of post-oncolytic tumor immunity in various inbred strains of mice. Although our findings are very preliminary, we present them here for the reader's interest. Table 15 summarizes our observations on the ability of several mouse strains to respond with anti-tumor antibody production following reovirus oncolysis of Sa 180.

All strains produced comparable titers (1:2000 to 1:10 000) of hemagglutinin-inhibiting anti-reovirus antibody during the experiment. This suggests that there is no major innate defect in the immunoglobulin synthesizing capacity of these strains. However, of 7 strains tested only 3 appeared capable of synthesizing an anti-tumor antibody detectable in serum by agglutination tests following oncolysis. These three (A2G, A/J, and C3H) are also strains which were passively protectable with A2G immune serum.

The four "non-responding" strains were strains which had been shown to be non-protectable passively with A2G immune serum. Mice of these strains usually succumbed to recurring ascites or subcutaneous tumors following reovirus oncolysis and were thus not available for challenge with tumor. In some experiments a reovirus oncolysate was used in attempts to immunize such mice. Both procedures failed to elicit anti-tumor agglutinin or anti-ε precipitin responses in these strains. F_1 offspring from crosses of non-protectable (RF) and protectable (A2G) mice did not respond with detectable agglutinin formation. Both ε-positive and ε-negative strains were represented among the "non-responders" while all responding strains were ε-negative.

h) Induction of Tumor Immunity Without Viral Oncolysis

Reports of successful immunization of mice against nonspecific tumors without viral oncolysis have appeared frequently in the literature (e. g. ANDERVONT, 1932; BESREDKA and GROSS, 1935; RÉVÉSZ, 1955; DONALDSON and MITCHELL, 1959; McKEE et al., 1959; BISMANIS, 1964; APFFEL et al., 1966). In none of these has the basis of such induced immunity been elucidated. What interested us most about experiments of this type was that they consistently reported failure to immunize with lysates obtained by mechanical disruption of tumor cells. This was true even when X-irradiated cells or alkylated cells could be shown to induce good immunity to the tumor in the mice used. Thus, APFFEL et al. (1966) were unable to induce immunity with EA lysates even though they used A/Jax mice, a strain which was immunizable in our hands.

If physical lysates of nonspecific tumor cells were *totally* non-immunogenic, then we might have to invoke some unusual hypothesis to explain the origin of the immunogen in the viral oncolysate. Perhaps we would have to postulate the induction of new cellular antigens by the oncolytic virus. This, however, seemed far-fetched since postoncolytic serum was perfectly capable of reacting with "normal" tumor cells which had not been exposed to the oncolytic agent.

To improve the sensitivity of the assay we used adjuvants and small challenge doses (KLEIN, 1965, and unpublished observations). Lysates of washed tumor cells were prepared by sonication or with the French press. Homogenates were either extracted with chloroform or left untreated, and adjusted to contain $1—2 \times 10^8$ EA cell equivalents per ml. These were then tested for their ability to actively immunize A2G mice against various challenge doses of the tumor. In all experiments the chloroform extracted and the untreated lysates were equally effective or ineffective in inducing such immunity. Mice surviving the primary challenge were re-challenged with higher doses of the tumor in all cases.

In all experiments each mouse received a total of 1×10^8 EA cell equivalents. This was given as a single injection or as several injections spaced at weekly intervals. Table 16 shows the result of an experiment using a chloroform extracted lysate.

Table 16. *Active Immunization of A2G Mice against Ehrlich Ascites Tumor with Physical Lysates of EA Tumor cells*

Type of immunization [a]	Challenge 1000 cells	Challenge 10^5 cells
EA lysate 1× i.p.	0/20 [b]	n. d. [c]
EA lysate 1× i.m. in Freund's complete adjuvant	0/20	n. d.
EA lysate 4× i.p.	1/10	n. d.
EA lysate 4× i.m.	1/10	n. d.
EA lysate 4× i.m. in Freund's complete adjuvant	21/27	1/8
Freund's complete adjuvant alone 4× i.m.	0/10	n. d.
None (control)	0/10	0/10

[a] Each injection contained the equivalent of 10^8 EA cells. The physical lysates were extracted with $CHCl_3$ and the aqueous phase used as a vaccine. Challenge inoculations were given 7 days after the last antigen injection.

[b] No. of mice protected / No. of mice in each group.

[c] n. d. = not done.

The lysate was relatively non-immunogenic when administered either once or four times intraperitoneally without adjuvant. The injection of the antigen one time with adjuvant or four times without adjuvant by the intramuscular route generally failed to induce tumor immunity in a significant proportion of the mice. However, most animals receiving the antigen four times in Freund's complete adjuvant sur-

Table 17. *Active Immunization of A2G Mice against Ehrlich Ascites Tumor with Physical Lysates of EA Tumor Cells Adsorbed to Bentonite*

Type of immunization [a]	Challenge 1000 cells
EA lysate 1× i.p.	0/12 [f]
EA lysate + bentonite 1× i.p. [b]	7/12
Supernatant from mixture of EA lysate + bentonite 1×i.p. [c]	0/12
Sediment from mixture of EA lysate + bentonite 1× i.p. [d]	7/11
Bentonite alone 1× i.p. [e]	0/12

[a] Each injection contained the equivalent of 1.5×10^8 EA cells. Challenge inoculations were given 15 days after antigen.

[b] EA lysate and bentonite pre-incubated for 2 hours on roller drum at 37° C. 10 mg of bentonite per injection.

[c] The mixture of EA lysate and bentonite pre-incubated as above was centrifuged at 20,000 g for 15 min.

[d] The pellet from the above centrifugation was resuspended in saline and injected at 10 mg of bentonite per injection.

[e] 10 mg of bentonite per injection.

[f] No. of mice protected / No. of mice in each group.

vived the primary challenge of 1000 cells (100 LD_{50}'s). Such mice were able to resist subsequent challenges with higher doses of the tumor. After several challenges, their sera could be shown to contain an agglutinin for tumor cells, an anti-ε precipitin, and a factor which protected A2G but not ICR mice against challenge with the tumor (KLEIN, 1965).

Ever since this finding, we have sought other ways in which the immunogenicity of non-specific tumor lysates might be demonstrated. DIETRICH (1964b), for example, reported that the absorption of an antigen to bentonite would greatly enhance its immunogenicity in C57Bl/6 mice. This idea sounded attractive and lead us to try similar experiments using the tumor lysate as the antigen (KLEIN, unpublished). Table 17 presents the results of an experiment of this type.

In this experiment each mouse received a total of 1.5×10^8 EA cell equivalents once intraperitoneally. The lysate again was quite ineffective as an inducer of tumor immunity when administered alone. However, the lysate proved to be effective when administered as a suspension containing bentonite particles. The bentonite particles which had been preincubated with the lysate were separated from the lysate by high speed centrifugation. The resultant supernatant when injected into mice had no immunogenic properties, whereas the resuspended washed bentonite pellet could immunize mice against the challenge tumor. Tests carried out on the supernatant revealed that the ε-alloantigen had been removed. We assume that it was adsorbed to the bentonite, but have no direct evidence for this at present.

Mice surviving multiple challenges of the tumor yielded sera with all of the measured properties of postoncolytic immune sera and "post-Freund's adjuvant" immune sera. This experiment demonstrated that a physical lysate of nonspecific tumor cells could be administered to immunocompetent mice a single time and elicit an immune response from a significant proportion of them. We might speculate and imagine that the adsorption of cellular antigens to virus particles is an important adjuvant factor during viral oncolysis. This would perhaps result in an enhanced uptake of antigen by phagocytic cells.

We have carried out several preliminary experiments to test the ability of homogenates of normal organs from various inbred strains of mice to immunize A2G mice against the EA tumor. We reasoned that certain strains might contain an antigen shared in common with the tumor cell. This assumption was based on our earlier observation of accelerated clearance of A2G anti-EA antibody in ICR mice, and on our experience that certain strains of mice could not be passively protected. We prepared aqueous extracts of the pooled livers, kidneys, and spleens from several strains. These were then administered to A2G mice with complete Freund's adjuvant. Table 18 records our results with this procedure.

Although larger numbers of animals must be utilized in future experiments, these results suggested that the immunization of mice against the EA tumor may be achieved with organ extracts of some non-protectable mouse strains. We have not yet checked the sera of these animals for immune globulin.

Since both the WSA influenza virus and reovirus type 3 attach to neuraminic-acid containing receptors (GOTTSCHALK, 1956; GOMATOS and TAMM, 1962) we thought that it might be interesting to see if preparations containing neuraminidase would in any way affect the immunogenicity of intact EA tumor cells (KLEIN, unpublished). We felt that this might provide some hint regarding the effectiveness of these viruses in inducing postoncolytic immunity. An experiment, again preliminary, is presented in Table 19. A cholera filtrate containing 1200 μg units of neuraminidase was utilized.

It is clear that the administration of between 150 μg and 600 μg neuraminidase activity prevented 4×10^6 EA cells (4×10^5 LD$_{50}$'s) from developing into tumor in most A2G mice. 75 μg of neuraminidase activity was ineffective in this respect.

Table 18. *Active Immunization of A2G Mice against Ehrlich Ascites Tumor with Aqueous Extracts of Normal Organs of Various Mouse Strains*

Type of immunization[a]	Challenge 1000 cells
ICR organ extract 4× i.m. in complete Freund's adjuvant	2/8 [b]
ICR serum 4× i.m. in complete Freund's adjuvant	0/6
RF organ extract 4× i.m. in complete Freund's adjuvant	2/6
RF serum 4× i.m. in complete Freund's adjuvant	0/6
AKR organ extract 4× i.m. in complete Freund's adjuvant	0/9
None (control)	0/10

    [a] Weekly injections, challenge 7 days after last injection.
    [b] No. of mice protected / No. of mice in each group.

Table 19. *Anti-tumor Immunity in A2G Mice Following Treatment of Ehrlich Ascites Tumor with Neuraminidase*

Description of experiment[a]	Outcome on day 33 [b]	Result of challenge with 5×10^4 EA cells[c]
4×10^6 EA cells + 600 units of neuraminidase	6/6	6/6
4×10^6 EA cells + 300 units of neuraminidase	6/6	3/6
4×10^6 EA cells + 150 units of neuraminidase	5/6	4/5
4×10^6 EA cells + 75 units of neuraminidase	0/6	—
4×10^6 EA cells alone	0/6	—

    [a] Washed tumor cells were inoculated together with the indicated amount of neuraminidase (filtrate of V. cholerae, Sigma Chemical Company) intraperitoneally on day 0. Survivors were challenged on day 33.
    [b] No. of mice without tumor on day 33 / No. of mice in each group.
    [c] No. of mice resisting challenge / No. of mice challenged.

Most mice surviving 33 days without evidence of tumor were able to resist subsequent challenge with 5000 LD$_{50}$'s. These mice contained in their serum both anti-ε precipitin and anti-EA agglutinin. We are quite aware that this does not constitute direct proof that it was indeed the neuraminidase in this filtrate which was the active factor in the filtrate and its identification as neuraminidase remains to be done.

V. General Discussion

We have proposed in the introduction to use our system of viral oncolysis as an exaggerated model of tumor-host relationships. The most perplexing feature of this relationship is the ability of tumors to grow from small inocula in spite of antigenic differences between tumor and host. Several possible explanations for this state of affairs have been mentioned in Chapter I: Weak antigenicity, resistance to the immune reaction, enhancement, tolerance, competition by host antigen. The hypothesis most commonly advanced to account for the growth of nonspecific tumors is the following: Such tumors do not differ fundamentally from strain-specific tumors. In particular, they do have a full set of histocompatibility antigens, but in reduced concentration. The low density of these antigens at the cell surface would be responsible for decreased immunogenicity, decreased vulnerability, and increased susceptibility to enhancement (HELLSTRÖM and MÖLLER, 1965).

Implicit in this concept, although not usually spelled out, is the idea that in those cases where immunity to such tumors *can* be demonstrated, the immunological attack is directed against classical histocompatibility targets. We do not know whether this indeed is the case in immunity induced by orthodox procedures, such as pre-treatment with heavily irradiated tumor cells or limited tumor growth followed by surgical excision. If this were so, it should be possible to establish the histocompatibility pattern of such venerable tumors as, for instance, the Ehrlich ascites tumor, thereby rehabilitating it as an object of serious study. This posthumous reconstruction of the genetic makeup of the mouse in which, under Paul Ehrlich's gaze, the tumor arose, should appeal to those with an inclination for immuno-archeology. To our knowledge, no such reconstruction has been presented as yet.

It proved impossible, however, to ascribe to classical histocompatibility antigens the very strong immunity observed as a result of viral oncolysis. We know very little about the distribution of our immunogen among different mouse strains. The immunogen was present in the three nonspecific tumors we have used. If we assume that the immunogen was absent from those mouse strains which could be passively protected against the tumor by postoncolytic serum (or which could be cured of the tumor by reovirus oncolysis), the pattern shown on Tables 10, 11 and 15 emerges. This list is too fragmentary to be suggestive of any close association between known histocompatibility factors and the immunogen in question. However, both protectable (C3H, CBA) and non-protectable (C58) mice were found within the same H-2 type. In addition, postoncolytic immune sera, although they powerfully agglutinated tumor cells, failed to agglutinate red blood cells from a number of mouse strains (PALM, personal communication).

We are on firmer ground in stating the non-identity of the ε-antigen with many of the known histocompatibility antigens. Since detection of ε in organ extracts is very easy, many strains could be screened. The distribution shown on Tables 4 and 6 clearly contradicts any association of ε with known H antigens. Physicochemical properties of ε distinguish it from H-2 antigenic preparations as far as present knowledge permits this conclusion.

Unfortunately, we are not in a position to state whether ε and the immunogen are identical. In fact, we have some evidence speaking against identity, such as failure to protect certain ε-negative strains (Table 11) and lack of immunogenicity of ε-rich fractions of viral oncolysates (Table 14). This negative evidence is not conclusive, and ε may yet turn out to be closely related to the immunogen. This view is substantiated by a certain correlation between protectability and absence of ε (Tables 10, 11), and by the finding that immunogenicity resides in extracts of tumor cells treated with chloroform, a chemical assault which probably leaves intact only antigens of a peculiar structure.

An unexpected difficulty which we have encountered involves the distinction between "strong" and "weak" antigens. Usually this difference is clear cut, because the strength of an antigen is expressed both by the ease with which it induces an immune response and by the effectiveness of such a response in rejecting the graft. Indeed it is customary to use this second effect as a measure of antigenic strength. If we apply this criterion, then both our immunogen and the ε-antigen are very strong antigens. It is difficult to imagine a stronger immunity than one which overcomes 10^6 LD_{50} of a rapidly growing tumor with ease and which can be passively transferred with a fraction of a drop of serum, or a better antibody response than one which manifests itself by visible precipitation. But these spectacular results were only obtained when viral oncolysis was used in the immunizing step. When growing undisturbed, the tumor behaved as if it were entirely non-immunogenic. More than 100 serial passages of the Ehrlich tumor in A2G mice neither reduced its susceptibility to the immune reaction nor its content in ε-antigen. Any immune response it may have evoked during its growth must have resulted in little immunoselective pressure. Cell-free tumor extracts were of such low immunogenicity that only repeated injections, the addition of adjuvants, and use of small challenges were able to reveal it (Tables 16 and 17). The virus, therefore, must have played an essential part in inducing postoncolytic immunity.

Adjuvant Effect of the Virus

If we look at our results in a naive and unprejudiced fashion, we might suspect that the virus exerted an adjuvant effect on the immunogenicity of an alloantigen in the tumor. How could such an adjuvant effect be explained?

It seems rather unlikely that the virus acted by its sole presence, such as might be the case with bentonite particles or killed bacteria added to an antigen. The mere admixture of egg-grown WSA virus to a physical lysate of tumor cells failed to increase its immunogenicity (LINDENMANN and KLEIN, in preparation). Another possibility would be that systemic viral infection increased *the host's* immunologic responsiveness, as has been observed with the lactic dehydrogenase virus (NOTKINS et al., 1966). This mechanism is also unlikely, since mice pre-immunized against the oncolytic virus could still be protected against the tumor with a viral oncolysate (LINDENMANN and KLEIN, in preparation).

We might simply suggest that viral oncolysis releases otherwise inaccessible immunogenic material. Lysis by physical means might either fail to liberate the antigen, or liberate it under circumstances where it is rapidly destroyed by cellular enzymes. Viral oncolysis could conceivably affect certain cellular structures and leave others intact. As a result, more of the immunogen could then be ingested by phagocytic cells, perhaps by a process similar to "piggyback" phagocytosis (SBARRA et al., 1962). Figure 22 shows whole chunks of virus-infected tumor cells being ingested by a macrophage. Unfortunately, we know too little on how the host handles physical lysates of tumor cells to interpret this finding.

It is known that influenza viruses incorporate host material, probably cell surface components, into their envelopes. Figures 6 and 7 are very suggestive in this respect.

Such incorporated material might show increased antigenicity [3]. It is, for instance, easier to produce antibodies to the host component of egg-grown influenza virus with infected allantoic fluid than with normal allantoic fluid, although the latter too contains the antigen (HARBOE, personal communication). Since oncolysis by reovirus, which has no envelope, resulted in much the same pattern of immunity, this possibility seems remote. Host material could be incorporated into the nucleoprotein of the virus — not a very appealing suggestion either, for the nucleoproteins of myxo- and reoviruses are very different. It is in general difficult to reconcile the idea of some specific viral action with the fact that viruses so distantly related as myxo- and reoviruses exert similar effects on the immunogen. Nevertheless, it is possible for even utterly unrelated viruses to produce indentical changes in host cells, for instance, to induce the synthesis of interferon.

Perhaps the important factor is not viral infection, but cell necrosis. Early investigators were impressed by the immunogenicity of tumors undergoing spontaneous or induced degeneration. CASPARI (1929) wrote: "Ich habe stets darauf hingewiesen, dass die besten Immunisierungen dann hervorgerufen werden, wenn lebende Zellen, speziell lebende Geschwulstzellen, im Organismus zugrunde gehen…".

A direct experimental proof of this concept was attempted by LEWIS and APTEK-MAN (1951). They ligated the vessels supplying large rat sarcomas and recovered the necrotic tumor masses after 2 to 4 days. These necrotic tissues were immunogenic when inoculated into other rats, whereas various homogenates or extracts from "healthy" tumors were not. Unfortunately, this line of work does not seem to have been pursued any further.

If we view the virus as an unspecific adjuvant, we are reminded of the possible adjuvant role of RNA in an early phase of the immune response (FISHMAN et al., 1965; ASKONAS and RHODES, 1965). It has been suggested that the function of the RNA might be to hold the antigen in native, immunogenic configuration (FRIEDMAN et. al., 1965). For instance, Turnip Yellow Mosaic Virus is a good antigen and readily induces antibodies directed against the viral protein, whereas the same protein stripped of its nucleic acid is a poor antigen (MARBROOK and MATTHEWS, 1966). We are far from understanding such phenomena fully. Some adjuvant effects of nucleic acids or oligonucleotides may be entirely nonspecific (MERRITT and JOHNSON, 1965), but this can hardly be an explanation for the action of a few drops of viral RNA added to the sea of cellular nucleic acid present in tumor lysates. It may be that in the turmoil produced by viral infection antigenic moieties become entangled with RNA of either viral or cellular origin and thus become potent antigens.

The host for some reason might be tolerant of the immunogen present in the tumor. DIETRICH (1964 a) has suggested that in this case breaking of tolerance should be attempted by chemical alterations of tumor cells. It seems possible that antigens altered by virus-induced enzymes or by incorporation into viral particles could

---

[3] Note added in proof: Since finishing this manuscript we have found some evidence pointing to a close association between the immunogen and the virus particles. Briefly, in mice pre-immunized with the virus the immunogenicity of viral oncolysates was enhanced. The addition of rabbit antiserum to egg grown virus, on the other hand, abolished the immunogenicity of viral oncolysates. Also, attempts at separating the immunogen from the virus particles have so far failed. (LINDENMANN and KLEIN, in preparation).

break tolerance. Alternatively, in the presence of the virus the antibody response could be shifted from one immunoglobulin class to another, thereby breaking a state of enhancement.

An obvious site of possible association between virus and cellular components of the tumor is the surface receptor. Neuraminidase removes receptors for both influenza virus and reovirus from red cells (GOMATOS and TAMM, 1962). Thus the two viruses which we have been using might have similar complementary structures by which they attach to tumor cells. Interaction of tumor cells and neuraminidase, which also has affinities to cell receptors of the two viruses, was indeed able to induce tumor immunity (Table 19). This work is still preliminary and much remains to be done, but a number of relatively simple experiments suggest themselves. For instance, tumor cells treated with neuraminidase and then lysed, or the cell-free supernatant of neuraminidase-treated tumor cells, could be tested for their immunizing power. BURNET and ANDERSON (1947) showed that treatment of red cells with Vibrio cholerae filtrate uncovered an antigen called "T" on the surface of the cells, and that the cell-free supernatant was able to induce the formation of anti-T antibodies.

Returning to the viral oncolysates, the physicochemical status of the immunogen could be directly approached by several fractionation procedures. Another oncolytic virus, such as West Nile, could be studied along similar lines. Incidentally, a better understanding of postoncolytic immunity might also shed light on the role of viral infections in autoimmune disorders. Much to our disappointment, we were unable to benefit from research done in this field. The relatively frequent neurological sequelae of the older techniques of rabies vaccination might have been related to an adjuvant effect of the virus, but we searched the literature in vain for a controlled test of this hypothesis [4].

Up to this point we have considered effects of viruses that are clearly oncolytic. Fortunately we are by no means restricted to such viruses. Non-oncolytic viruses may well have similar effects on the immunogenicity of tumor cells. This is indicated by a report from BIGGS and EISELEIN (1965), who showed that a tumor spontaneously infected with some non-oncolytic passenger virus was immunogenic when implanted in a diffusion chamber. The immunity induced in this case seemed to be directed mainly against the infected tumor line and not against its non-infected counterpart. It would be very important to distinguish in similar situations between enhanced immunogenicity of pre-existing antigens and induction of neoantigens by the virus. Svet-Moldavsky has suggested that "artifical heterogenization" of tumors by non-oncolytic viruses such as polyoma might induce the formation of targets suitable for immunological attack (SVET-MOLDAVSKY and HAMBURG, 1964; HAMBURG and SVET-MOLDAVSKI, 1964).

The possibilities become really staggering if we realize that not only viruses, but probably any type of intracellular parasite could have similar effects. Thus, a sporo-

---

[4] Note added in proof: Schwentker and Rivers have shown that antibodies to brain could be induced in rabbits by injecting them with autolysed or vaccinia-infected brain tissue (SCHWENTKER, F. F., and T. M. RIVERS: The antibody response of rabbits to injections of emulsions and extracts from homologous brain. J. exp. Med. 60, 559 (1934)). The possible role of viruses in initiation of autoimmune disorders has been recently discussed by PETTE et al. (Ann. N. Y. Acad. Sci. 122, 417 (1965)), VAN LOGHEM (Vox Sang. 10, 1 (1965)) and DAMESHEK (Lancet 1966/i, 1268).

zoon found in a Yoshida sarcoma induced regression of the tumor in a number of cases, whereupon the survivors were immune to challenge with the non-infected tumor (PETRI, 1966). Several reports on the effects of trypanosomes, bacteria, toxins, etc. should be reconsidered in this light. Finally, since any effects observed in biological systems must be mediated by the interactions of certain substances, chemical manipulations of tumors to render them more immunogenic should be attempted. We have already mentioned neuraminidase as a promising agent. Alkylation of tumor cells as used by APFFEL et al. (1966) is perhaps another way of achieving a similar result [5]. The range of possible chemicals is almost limitless.

We have always insisted on regarding viral oncolysis as a model. This model, in turn, is susceptible of being studied with the help of another model, a model of the model, so to speak. BARTELL et al. (1963) reported that 5 to 21 days after mice had been cured of a staphylococcal infection with a specific phage, the animals were immune to large challenges with the staphylococcus. It is difficult to judge from this report how easily the same degree of immunity could have been attained by other means. Similar experiments should be done with systems in which good immunity is notoriously difficult to achieve, such as infection of mice with Salmonella typhimurium. Cure of the infection with an appropriate bacteriophage might lead to solid immunity.

Status of the Antigens Uncovered by Viral Oncolysis

How should we interpret, classify, call the antigens uncovered by viral oncolysis? One of the difficulties here is that the number of antigens involved is unknown. The antigens are recognized with the aid of immune reactions — the immunogen by the immunity it induces, the agglutinogen by agglutination, the ε-antigen by precipitation with antiserum. The three may be different, or they may be the same. We know the ε-antigen best, for technical reasons, and shall therefore discuss the other two only briefly.

We are totally ignorant of the role these antigens play in the normal economy of the cell. The agglutinogen is probably located near the surface. The immunogen must be a sensitive target for immune attack. The ε-antigen must have persisted for innumerable transfer generations in some tumors. An antigen cross-reacting with anti-ε antibody seems to be almost universally distributed among mammalian species (Table 8). Yet A2G mice seem to be doing very well without it. Could these antigens be footprints left behind by passenger viruses? With long-transplanted tumors this

---

[5] Note added in proof: Two more papers from this group of workers have come to our attention: In one, they state that cell-free fluid from several tumors could be rendered immunogenic by treatment with iodo-acetate (APFFEL, C. A., and B. G. ARNASON: Immunization with sulfhydryl-alkylated tumor material. Proc. Am. Ass. Cancer Res. 7, 3 (1966)). In the other, they are apparently able to do the same thing with untreated cell-free ascitic fluid (APFFEL, C. A., B. G. ARNASON, C. W. TWINAM, and C. A. HARRIS: Recovery with immunity after serial tapping of transplantable mouse ascites tumors. Brit. J. Cancer 20, 122 (1966)). An interesting point about this report is the observation that in the tumors used, 40% of the cells present on the 16th day of tumor growth appeared to be inflammatory cells. One wonders if this does not reflect infection of the tumor by some oncolytic agent, so that the immunities observed would be actually cases of postoncolytic immunity.

could very well be the case. However, the presence of ε in many mouse strains and its mode of inheritance (Table 5) argue strongly against this possibility.

The ε-antigen, then, is an alloantigen, or, by the nomenclature favored until recently, an isoantigen. Can this antigen be called a transplantation antigen? Certainly ε is not one of the antigens whose distribution is easily studied by classical transplantation methods, otherwise it would have been discovered long ago. Mice carrying ε and mice lacking it have been used extensively in transplantation studies without its existence being suspected. If under "normal" transplantation conditions ε is an extremely weak antigen, then the issue will only be settled by the development of congenic strains, one with, the other without ε. We, for our part, believe that it is entirely possible for ε to be a cellular alloantigen which does not induce an immune response upon ordinary transplantation. Such an antigen should probably not be called a transplantation antigen, even if it can be shown that an immune reaction mounted against it results in graft rejection.

However, this is a field in which we feel even less at home than in the others. We therefore propose to leave the matter open until the antigens concerned will have been studied by workers more familiar with transplantation immunology. This is the reason for our provisional nomenclature, which uses a Greek letter for the best defined of our antigens and leaves the others (if indeed there are others) anonymous. It is surprising that cellular alloantigenic differences between strains of mice have not been revealed by precipitation before. Alloantigenic precipitating serum components are, of course, well recognized, including components governed by H-2 alleles (SCHREFFLER, 1964). Since mice have a reputation of being poor producers of precipitating antibody (AMOS, 1959), this may be a reason. HIRAI (1965) has recently found a cellular alloantigen of rats by precipitation. In man, evidence has been obtained for the existence of pancreas-specific precipitating alloantigens, although the antisera used were of xenogeneic origin (METZGAR, 1964).

Transplantation immunologists have been extremely inventive in the range of procedures used to detect immunity once it is induced. The methodology ranges from simple agglutination to sophisticated tracer techniques. Compared with this, the methods used for inducing transplantation immunity seem to have stagnated. Tissue transplantation, tumor growth followed by spontaneous regression or surgical excision, injection of cells or cell homogenates, treatment with X-irradiated tumor cells have all been popular for more than 50 years. Less conventional techniques have been used only sporadically, among others, intracaecal inoculation (LUND, 1957), pretreatment with cultivated cells of reduced virulence (HSU, 1960), immunization with Streptomycin complexes (POLGLASE, 1963). It might be worth while for transplantation immunologists to look into some of the approaches to immunization suggested in the preceding section.

Mechanism of Postoncolytic Immunity

One of the most unexpected findings during our work was the effectiveness of postoncolytic serum in passive transfer of immunity. STUART and EL HASSAN (1964) experienced a similar surprise when studying the passive transfer of immunity to the Landschütz ascites tumor. Passive immunization could also be achieved adoptively by the transfer of syngeneic lymphoid cells, but the existence of a strong humoral immunity made it difficult to evaluate the possible participation of purely cellular immunity (BOYSE et al., 1962). The immune serum did not seem to act directly on the cells, for evidence of rapid cytolysis was obtained neither *in vivo* nor *in vitro*. Rather, the antibody induced aggregations of host cells around tumor cells (Figure 16). The tumor ceased to grow in the presence of antibody (Figure 15 a), yet occasional mitoses were seen. We have to assume that for every tumor cell undergoing mitosis in the presence of antibody, a tumor cell disappeared, at least during the first 80 hours of antiserum action. Eventually, more tumor cells must have been destroyed than were continually being formed. It may be that interphase cells were more or less protected against immunological attack, but that mitosis represented a phase of increased vulnerability. Quantitative determinations of the mitotic index were not performed, but would be of obvious value.

How did the antibody induce the aggregation of host cells around tumor cells? Union of antibody and antigen might have released chemotactic substances which attracted host cells, or the antibody might have stuck first to the host cells and might have then attached the host cells to their tumor targets. This mechanism would involve a double affinity of the antibody for host cells and tumor cells. The affinity for host cells might be relatively nonspecific (akin to cytophilic antibody) or might actually represent serologic cross-reaction between an antigen on tumor cells and a related antigen on host cells. The opsonizing effect of isoantiserum directed against both host macrophages and tumor cells has been demonstrated by BENNETT and LICURSI (1964).

Antibody could protect only certain strains of mice and not others. Possible mechanisms were discussed in Chapter IV, section e (p. 45). We favor the hypothesis that those strains of mice which could not be protected shared an antigen related to the immunogen on the tumor, and absorbed the antibody. The same mouse strains which were passively protectable should prove actively immunizable by oncolysis or with an oncolysate. It should be noted, however, that the barrier to passive protection was not absolute. Thus, the tumor seemed perfectly controlled during the first 24 hours after serum administration in both protectable and non-protectable mice. The successful protection of "non protectable" mice may be a matter of dosage or repeated injections. Antiserum given protectable mice was not only effective when administred along with the tumor, but could be given up to 4 days after the tumor (LINDENMANN, unpublished). Here again, the quantity of antibody must have been an important factor, and it is possible that more antibody would be effective even if applied later.

At the beginning of our work we felt strongly handicapped by the necessity of using A2G mice to the exclusion of any other mouse strain. This limitation was imposed upon us by the genetic resistance of A2G mice to influenza virus (see Chapter III). In one of the delightful oddities that make the charm of scientific research it now turns out that this was an extraordinarily happy choice, since A2G mice belong to the few strains that are easily protectable. We do not wish to suggest that other strains will not prove to be protectable after all, but chances are that the effects will be more borderline and less dramatic.

Possible Human Applications

The temptation to speculate on possible applications of our findings to medicine is too strong to resist. Oncolysis proper has been tried out on human beings, with results that were not encouraging (SOUTHAM, 1960). In a recent clinical trial WEBB et al. (1966) treated 28 patients with advanced leukemia and other malignancies with two arboviruses. In no case was there any question of a patient being cured. However, four patients were thought to have definitely benefited from the treatment. In discussing possible beneficial effects of viral treatment on tumors, WEBB et al. considered 3 mechanisms:

a) Oncolysis proper.

b) Interference with an oncogenic virus, induction of interferon.

c) Enhancement of antigenicity of tumor cells.

The first mechanism has served as a theoretical basis for most oncolysis experiments performed in the past. Its successful application to man meets formidable obstacles. The second mechanism was the leading idea behind the therapeutic trial reported by WHEELOCK and DINGLE (1964), who repeatedly administered large doses of several viruses to a patient with acute leukemia and noted a number of remissions. Therapeutic efforts inspired by the third mechanism have, to our knowledge, not yet been reported. It is this mechanism which offers perhaps the best prospects.

For such an approach to be feasible, the following highly hypothetical conditions should be fulfilled: The tumor to be treated should possess vulnerable antigenic targets, and the host should be able to respond to adequate antigenic stimulation. A virus capable of growing in the tumor and of greatly enhancing the antigenicity of its antigen(s) would then have to be found. Oncolysis need not be performed *in vivo*. Indeed, it would be advantageous to grow the tumor, for instance, by an organ culture technique of the type recently employed by DICKSON (1966), or at least to maintain surviving fragments of it *in vitro*. "Oncolysis" would take place *in vitro*, and the oncolysate could be used as a vaccine to immunize the patient.

Needless to say, these are wild speculations resting on shaky premises. However, rather than being pessimistic and pointing out the various difficulties ahead, which others undoubtedly will do, we prefer to stress some interesting possibilities. Many more viruses could be used than with straightforward oncolysis, including highly virulent strains or viruses against which immunity is widespread. With pathogenic viruses, suitable means of inactivating them without harming the tumor antigen might be found. Alternately, the patient might be first immunized against the virus, a procedure which in mice does not impair the immunogenicity of viral oncolysates (LINDENMANN and KLEIN, in preparation). For the same reason, viruses against which the patient is naturally immune could be employed. The list of candidate viruses becomes almost endless, and more than one virus may be useful, so that the chances of rapidly finding a virus suitable for a given tumor would be correspondingly increased. With accumulating experience, a bank of potent antigens could be set up covering the spectrum of the more widely distributed tumors.

Just to show the technical feasibility of such an approach, we have actually cultivated tumor cells from a moribund cancer patient, have infected these *in vitro* with a strain of fowl plague virus previously adapted to HeLa and KB cells, and have used the resulting oncolysate as a vaccine for the patient (LINDENMANN and

STORCK, unpublished). It would be premature to report any clinical details, and we prefer to return to our experimental model in order to learn more about it. Should this booklet entice others to join the field of postoncolytic immunity, we would feel amply rewarded for our efforts.

Summary

Three brief reviews on tumor immunology, viral oncolysis and inborn resistance of mice to viruses introduce a description of the following experimental model. A2G mice, which are naturally resistant to myxoviruses, are inoculated with a non-specific ascites tumor. Several days later oncolysis is induced by infection of the tumor with a tumor-adapted strain of influenza virus, WSA. Mice surviving oncolysis are solidly immune to challenge with several nonspecific ascites tumors.

This immunity is mediated by circulating antibodies. It can be passively transferred to certain inbred mouse strains, but not to others. The sera of immune mice regularly contain an agglutinin for tumor cells and frequently a precipitin which reacts with aqueous extracts of certain mouse tumors and of normal organs from a number of mouse strains. The alloantigen responsible for this reaction is called ε. The relationship between immunogen, agglutinogen and ε-alloantigen and its bearing on the passive protectability of mice are discussed. Known histocompatibility antigens do not seem to be involved in any of these reactions.

When oncolysis is performed in one set of mice and the virus-infected tumor is removed after 2—3 days and homogenized, the homogenate injected into another set of mice of a suitable strain readily induces solid immunity. Similar homogenates from non-infected tumors are only very weakly immunogenic. The ways in which the virus might exert an adjuvant effect on alloantigens present in the tumor are discussed.

The main features of oncolysis and postoncolytic immunity induced by influenza virus can be reproduced with another, unrelated oncolytic agent, reovirus 3.

Possible applications to medicine are briefly considered.

Acknowledgements: We thank Mrs. M. Acklin and Miss A. Brunet for excellent technical assistance and Miss M. Schaich for help in preparing the manuscript.

References

ABELEV, G. I., S. D. PEROVA, N. I. KHRAMKOVA, Z. A. POSTNIKOVA, and I. S. IRLIN: Production of embryonal α-globulin by transplantable mouse hepatomas. Transplantation 1, 174 (1963).

ABERCROMBIE, M., and E. J. AMBROSE: The surface properties of cancer cells: A review. Cancer Res. 22, 525 (1962).

ACKERMANN, W. W., and H. KURTZ: A new host-virus system. Proc. Soc. exp. Biol. (N. Y.) 81, 421 (1952).

ALLISON, A. C.: Genetic factors in resistance against virus infections. Arch. Virusforsch. 17, 280 (1965).

AMOS, D. B.: The persistence of mouse iso-antibodies in vivo. Brit. J. Cancer 9, 216 (1955).

— Some iso-antigenic system of the mouse. Canad. Cancer Conf. 3, 241 (1959).

Amos, D. B.: The use of simplified systems as an aid to the interpretation of mechanisms of graft rejection. Progr. Allergy 6, 468 (1962).
— Transplantation antigens in mouse, rat and man. Progr. med. Genet. 3, 106 (1964).
—, M. Zumpft, and P. Armstrong: H-5.A and H-6.A, two mouse isoantigens on red cells and tissues detected serologically. Transplantation 1, 270 (1963).
Andervont, H. B.: Studies on immunity induced by mouse sarcoma 180. Publ. Hlth Rep. 47, 1859 (1932).
Andrews, P.: Estimation of the molecular weights of proteins by Sephadex gel-filtration. Biochem. J. 91, 222 (1964).
— The gel-filtration behavior of proteins related to their molecular weights over a wide range. Biochem. J. 96, 595 (1965).
Apffel, C. A., B. G. Arnason, and J. H. Peters: Induction of tumour immunity with tumour cells treated with iodoacetate. Nature (Lond.) 209, 694 (1966).
Askonas, B. A., and J. M. Rhodes: Is antigen associated with macrophage RNA? Molecular and Cellular Basis of Antibody Formation (J. Sterzl, Ed.) 503. Publishing House of the Czechoslovak Ac. Sc., Prague 1965.
Banfield, W. G., P. A. Woke, C. M. MacKay, and H. L. Cooper: Mosquito transmission of a reticulum cell sarcoma of hamsters. Science 148, 1239 (1965).
Bang, F. B., and A. Warwick: Mouse macrophages as host cells for the mouse hepatitis virus and the genetic basis of their susceptibility. Proc. Nat. Acad. Sci. 46, 1065 (1960).
Bartell, P. F., I. S. Thind, T. Orr, and W. S. Blakemore: The in vivo interaction between staphylococcus bacteriophage and Staphylococcus aureus. J. exp. Med. 118, 13 (1963).
Bayreuther, K.: Der Chromosomenbestand des Ehrlich-Ascites-Tumors der Maus. Z. Naturforsch. 7 B, 554 (1952).
Bennett, B.: Specific suppression of tumor growth by isolated peritoneal macrophages from immunized mice. J. Immunol. 95, 656 (1965).
—, and P. Licursi: Action of isoimmune serum on peritoneal cells in vitro. Proc. Soc. exp. Biol. (N. Y.) 116, 404 (1964).
Bennette, J. G.: Isolation of a non-pathogenic tumor destroying virus from mouse ascites. Nature (Lond.) 187, 72 (1960).
Besredka, A., and L. Gross: De l'immunisation contre le sarcome de la souris par la voie intracutanée. Ann. Inst. Pasteur 55, 491 (1935).
Biggs, M. W., and J. E. Eiselein: Diffusion chamber studies of allogenic tumor immunity in mice. Cancer Res. 25, 1888 (1965).
Billingham, R. E., L. Brent, and P. B. Medawar: Actively acquired tolerance of foreign cells. Nature 172, 603 (1953).
Bismanis, J. E.: Immunization of mice against Ehrlich ascites carcinoma with formalinised tumour cells grown in tissue culture. J. Path. Bact. 87, 444 (1964).
Bloch, K. J.: Heterogeneity in biologic functions of antibodies: implications for immunologic tumor enhancement. Fed. Proc. 24, 1030 (1965).
Boone, C., M. Sasaki, and R. W. McKee: Characterization of an in vitro strain of Ehrlich-Lettré ascites carcinoma subjected to many periodic mouse passages. J. Nat. Cancer Inst. 34, 725 (1965).
Bower, B. F., and G. S. Gordon: Hormonal effects of nonendocrine tumors. Ann. Rev. Med. 16, 83 (1965).
Boyden, S. V.: Cellular discrimination between indigenous and foreign matter. J. theoret. Biol. 3, 123 (1962 a).
— The chemotactic effect of mixtures of antibody and antigens on polymorphonuclear leucocytes. J. exp. Med. 115, 453 (1962 b).
Boyle, W., D. A. L. Davies, and G. Haughton: Mouse tissue cell antigens. Some properties of cell-bound components. Immunology 6, 499 (1963).
Boyse, E. A., L. J. Old, and E. Stockert: Some further data on cytotoxic isoantibodies in the mouse. Ann. N. Y. Acad. Sci. 99, 574 (1962).
Briody, B. A., and W. A. Cassel: Adaptation of influenza virus to mice. II. Changes in the growth curve of an A prime stain of influenza virus. J. Immunol. 74, 37 (1955).

BRIODY, B. A., W. A. CASSEL, J. LYTLE, and M. FEARING: Adaptation of influenza virus to mice. I. Genetic and environmental factors affecting an A prime strain of influenza virus. Yale J. Biol. Med. **25**, 391 (1953).

BROOME, J. D.: Evidence that the L-asparaginase of guinea pig serum is responsible for its antilymphoma effects. J. exp. Med. **118**, 99 (1963).

BURNET, F. M., and S. G. ANDERSON: The "T" antigen of guinea-pig and human red cells. Austr. J. exp. Biol. **25**, 213 (1947).

CARTER, S. B.: Principles of cell motility. Nature (Lond.) **208**, 1183 (1966).

CASPARI, W.: Die experimentale Erforschung der Geschwülste vom Standpunkt der Infektions- und Immunitätslehre. Handb. Path. Mikroorg. Bd. 1 Teil 2, 1225. 3. Aufl. (1929).

CASSEL, W. A.: Multiplication of influenza virus in the Ehrlich ascites carcinoma. Cancer Res. **17**, 618 (1957).

—, and R. E. GARRETT: Newcastle disease virus as an antineoplastic agent. Cancer **18**, 86 (1965).

CHANG, S.-S., and W. H. HILDEMANN: Inheritance of susceptibility to polyoma virus in mice. J. Nat. Cancer Inst. **33**, 303 (1964).

CINADER, B., and S. DUBISKI: Effect of autologous protein on the specificity of the antibody response: Mouse and rabbit antibody to MuBl. Nature (Lond.) **202**, 102 (1964).

— —, and A. C. WARDLAW: Distribution, inheritance, and properties of an antigen, MuBl, and its relation to hemolytic complement. J. exp. Med. **120**, 897 (1964).

COHEN, E. P., R. W. NEWCOMB, and L. K. CROSBY: Conversion of nonimmune spleen cells to antibody-forming cells by RNA: strain specificity of the response. J. Immunol. **95**, 583 (1965).

COHN, Z. A.: The fate of bacteria within phagocytic cells. III. Destruction of an *Escherichia coli* agglutinogen within polymorphonuclear leucocytes and macrophages. J. exp. Med. **120**, 869 (1963).

Committee on standardized genetic nomenclature for mice: Standardized nomenclature for inbred strains of mice. Second listing. Cancer Res. **20**, 145 (1960).

COOPER, H. L., C. M. MACKAY, and W. G. BANFIELD: Chromosome studies of a contagious reticulum cell sarcoma of the Syrian hamster. J. Nat. Cancer Inst. **33**, 691 (1964).

DAMESHEK, W.: Autoimmunity: theoretical aspects. Ann. N. Y. Acad. Sci. **124**, 6 (1965).

DAVIES, D. A. L.: The isolation of mouse antigens carrying H-2 histocompatibility specificity: Some preliminary studies. Biochem. J. **84**, 307 (1962).

DICKSON, J. A.: Tissue culture approach to the treatment of cancer. Brit. Med. J. 1966/i, 817.

DIETRICH, F. M.: Immunologische Toleranz. Schweiz. med. Wschr. **94**, 109 (1964 a).

— Antikörperbildung gegen lösliche, aggregierte, praezipitierte und adsorbierte Proteine in C57BL/6-Mäusen. Pathol. Microbiol. **27**, 356 (1964 b).

DONALDSON, D. M., and J. R. MITCHELL: Immunization against Ehrlich ascites carcinoma with X-irradiated tumor cells. Proc. Soc. exp. Biol. (N. Y.) **101**, 204 (1959).

EATON, M. D., J. D. LEVINTHAL, A. R. SCALA, and M. L. JEWELL: Immunity and antibody formation induced by intraperitoneal or subcutaneous injection of Krebs-2 ascites tumor cells treated with influenza virus. J. Nat. Cancer Inst. **34**, 661 (1965).

EDWARDS, J. L., A. L. KOCH, P. YOUCIS, H. L. FREESE, M. B. LAITE, and J. T. DONALSON: Some characteristics of DNA synthesis and the mitotic cycle in Ehrlich ascites tumor cells. J. Biophys. Biochem. Cytol. **7**, 273 (1960).

FAHEY, J, L., J. WUNDERLICH, and R. MISHELL: The immunoglobulins of mice. I. Four major classes of immunoglobulins: $7S\gamma_2$-, $7S\gamma_1$-, $\gamma1A$ $(\beta2A)$-, and $18S\gamma1M$-globulins. J. exp. Med. **120**, 223 (1964).

FELDMAN, M., and L. SACHS: Immunogenetic properties of tumors that have acquired homo-transplantability. J. Nat. Cancer Inst. **20**, 513 (1958).

FISHMAN, M., and F. L. ADLER: Antibody formation initiated *in vitro*. II. Antibody synthesis in x-irradiated recipients of diffusion chambers containing nucleic acid derived from marcrophages incubated with antigen. J. exp. Med. **117**, 595 (1963).

—, J. J. Van ROOD, and F. L. ADLER: The initiation of antibody formation by ribonucleic acid from specifically stimulated macropages. Molecular and Cellular Basis of Antibody Formation (J. STERZL, Ed.) 491. Publishing House of the Czechoslovak Academy of Sciences, Prague 1965.

Flanagan, A. D., R. Love, and W. Tesar: Propagation of Newcastle disease virus in Ehrlich ascites cells in vitro and in vivo. Proc. Soc. exp. Biol. (N. Y.) 90, 82 (1955).

Francis, T. Jr., and A. E. Moore: A study of the neurotropic tendency in strains of the virus of epidemic influenza. J. exp. Med. 72, 717 (1940).

Freund, J.: The mode of action of immunologic adjuvants. Adv. Tuberc. Res. 7, 130 (1956).

Friedman, H. P., A. B. Stavitsky, and J. M. Solomon: Induction in vitro of antibodies to phage T2: Antigens in the RNA extracts employed. Science 149, 1106 (1965).

Furusawa, E., and W. Cutting: Propagation of Columbia SK virus in Ehrlich ascites tumor cells with oncolysis. Proc. Soc. exp. Biol. (N. Y.) 103, 618 (1960).

Gallily, R., A. Warwick, and F. B. Bang: Effect of cortisone on genetic resistance to mouse hepatitis virus in vivo and in vitro. Proc. Nat. Acad. Sci. 51, 1158 (1964).

Gill, F. A., and R. M. Cole: The fate of a bacterial antigen (streptococal M protein) after phagocytosis by macrophages. J. Immunol. 94, 898 (1965).

Ginder, D. R., and W. F. Friedewald: Effect of Semliki forest virus on rabbit fibromas. Proc. Soc. exp. Biol. (N. Y.) 77, 272 (1951).

Ginsburg, H., and L. Sachs: Destruction of mouse and rat embryo cells in tissue culture by lymph nodes from unsensitized rats. J. cell., comp. Physiol. 66, 199 (1965).

Gold, P., and O. Freedman: Specific carcinoembryonic antigens of the human digestive system. J. exp. Med. 122, 467 (1965).

Gomatos, P. J., and I. Tamm: Reactive sites of reovirus type 3 and their interaction with receptor substances. Virology 17, 455 (1962).

Goodman, G. T., and H. Koprowski: Study of the mechanism of innate resistance to virus infection. J. cell. comp. Physiol. 59, 333 (1962).

Gottschalk, A.: The influenza virus enzyme and its mucoprotein substrate. Yale J. Biol. Med. 26, 352 (1956).

Gowans, J. L., and D. D. McGregor: The immunological activities of lymphocytes. Progr. Allergy 9, 1 (1965).

— —, D. M. Cowen, and C. E. Ford: Initiation of immune responses by small lymphocytes. Nature (Lond.) 196, 651 (1962).

Gowen, J. W.: Genetic effects in nonspecific resistance to infectious disease. Bact. Reviews 24, 192 (1960).

Granger, G. A., and R. S. Weiser: Homograft target cells: Contact destruction in vitro by immune macrophages. Science 151, 97 (1966).

Gröschel, D., and H. Koprowski: Development of a virus-resistant inbred mouse strain for the study of innate resistance to Arbo B viruses. Arch. Virusforsch. 17, 379 (1965).

Grumbach, A.: Zur Bakteriologie des BCG. Schweiz. Med. Wschr. 86, 1159 (1956).

Habel, K.: Resistance of polyoma virus immune animals to transplanted polyoma tumors. Proc. Soc. exp. Biol. (N. Y.) 106, 722 (1961).

Hallauer, C.: Über das Verhalten von Hühnerpestvirus in der Gewebekultur. Z. Hyg. Infektionskrank. 113, 61 (1931).

Hamburg, V. P., and G. J. Svet-Moldavsky: Artificial heterogenization of tumours by means of Herpes simplex and polyoma viruses. Nature (Lond.) 203, 772 (1964).

Hartley, J. W., W. P. Rowe, and R. J. Huebner: Recovery of reoviruses from wild and laboratory mice. Proc. Soc. exp. Biol. (N. Y.) 108, 390 (1961).

Hartveit, F.: The significance of the blood content of the Ehrlich ascites carcinoma. Brit. J. Cancer 15, 665 (1961).

Haughton, G.: Naturally occurring soluble H-2 specificity in mouse tissues. Immunology 9, 193 (1965).

Hauschka, T. S.: Correlation of chromosomal and physiologic changes in tumors. J. cell. comp. Physiol. 52 suppl. 1, 197 (1958).

—, and A. Levan: Cytologic and functional characterization of single cell clones isolated from the Krebs-2 and Ehrlich ascites tumors. J. Nat. Cancer Inst. 21, 77 (1958).

Hellström, K. E., and G. Möller: Immunological and immunogenetic aspects of tumor transplantation. Progr. Allergy 9, 158 (1965).

—, I. Hellström, and C. Bergheden: Allogeneic inhibition of tumour cells by *in vitro* contact with cells containing foreign H-2 antigens. Nature (Lond.) 208, 458 (1965).

HERZENBERG, L. A., N. L. WARNER, and L. A. HERZENBERG: Immunoglobulin isoantigens (allotypes) in the mouse. I. Genetics and cross-reactions of the 7Sγ2A-isoantigens controlled by alleles at the IG-1 locus. J. exp. Med. 121, 415 (1965).

HIRAI, H.: Isoprecipitin in the sera of rats resistant to tumour transplantation. Nature (Lond.) 208, 798 (1965).

HOLMES, F. O.: Genetics of pathogenicity in viruses and of resistance in host plants. Adv. Virus Res. 11, 139 (1965).

HOTCHIN, J. E., S. M. COHEN, H. RUSKA, and C. RUSKA: Electron microscopical aspects of hemadsorption in tissue cultures infected with influenza virus. Virology 6, 689 (1958).

HOTZ, G., and W. SCHÄFER: Ultrahistologische Studie über die Vermehrung des Virus der klassischen Geflügelpest. Ztschr. Naturforsch. 10 B, 1 (1955).

HSÜ, L.-C., H.-S. YÜ, W.-S. CH'I, and C.-Y. TS'AO: Marker chromosomes of Ehrlich ascites carcinoma. Chinese Med. J. 83, 32 (1964).

HSU, T. C.: Reduction of transplantability of Novikoff hepatoma cells grown in vitro and the consequent protecting effect to the host against their malignant progenitor. J. Nat. Cancer Inst. 25, 927 (1960).

JAHKOLA, M.: Nature and inheritance of the resistance of inbred mice to tumor induction by polyoma virus. Acta path. microbiol. scand. suppl. 173, 1 (1965).

JONSSON, N., and H. O. SJÖGREN: Specific teransplantation immunity in relation to Rous sarcoma virus tumorigenesis in mice. J. exp. Med. 123, 487 (1966).

JOURNEY, L. J., and D. B. AMOS: An electron microscope study of histiocyte response to ascites tumor homograft. Cancer Res. 22, 998 (1962).

KAHAN, B. D.: Isolation of a soluble transplantation antigen. Proc. Nat. Acad. Sci. 53, 153 (1965).

KALISS, N.: Immunological enhancement and inhibition of tumor growth: Relationship to various immunological mechanisms. Fed. Proc. 24, 1024 (1965).

KANDUTSCH, A. A., and J. H. STIMPFLING: Partial purification of tissue isoantigens from a mouse sarcoma. Transplantation 1, 201 (1963).

KANTOCH, M., A. WARWICK, and F. B. BANG: The cellular nature of genetic susceptibility to a virus. J. exp. Med. 117, 781 (1963).

KATO, N., A. OKADA, and H. HARA: Early pulmonary lesion in the CFW strain mice produced by intravenous injection of influenza virus. Jap. J. Microbiol. 5, 283 (1961).

KAZIWARA, K.: Derivation of stable polyploid sublines from a hyperdiploid Ehrlich ascites carcinoma. Cancer Res. 14, 795 (1954).

KLEIN, G., H. O. SJÖGREN, and E. KLEIN: Demonstration of host resistance against sarcomas induced by implantation of cellophane films in isologous (syngeneic) recipients. Cancer Res. 23, 84 (1963).

— — —, and K. E. HELLSTRÖM: Demonstration of resistance against methylcholanthrene induced sarcomas in the primary autochthonous host. Cancer Res. 20, 1561 (1960).

KLEIN, P. A.: Immunization against the Ehrlich ascites carcinoma with a water soluble antigen. Fed. Proc. 24, 697 (1965).

—, and J. LINDENMANN: Further studies on the soluble ε-antigen of the mouse. Pathol. Microbiol. 28, 698 (1965).

KOCH, M. A., and A. B. SABIN: Specificity of virus-induced resistance to transplantation of polyoma and SV 40 tumors in adult hamsters. Proc. Soc. exp. Biol. (N. Y.) 113, 4 (1963).

KOPROWSKA, I., and H. KOPROWSKI: Morphologic and biologic changes in a mouse ascites tumor following induced infection with certain viruses. Cancer Res. 13, 651 (1953).

KOPROWSKI, H.: Ascites tumors as culture media in quantitative growth studies of viral agents. Ann N. Y. Acad. Sci. 63, 895 (1956).

—, and R. LOVE: The effect of virus infections upon ascites tumors of mice. Proc. Am. Ass. Cancer Res. 1, 30 (1953).

— —, and I. KOPROWSKA: Enhancement of susceptibility to viruses in neoplastic tissues. Texas Rep. Biol. Med. 15, 559 (1957).

KRULWICH, T. A., C. F. JACOBS, J. H. WEISMAN, and C. M. SOUTHAM: Studies of six new viruses in tumor-bearing mice. Cancer Res. 22, 322 (1962).

LAW, L. W.: Thymus: Role of resistance to polyoma virus oncogenesis. Science 147, 164 (1965).

LETTRÉ, H.: Einige Beobachtungen über das Wachstum des Mäuse-Ascites-Tumors und seine Beeinflussung. Hoppe-Seyler's Z. **268**, 59 (1941).

LEVADITI, C., and P. HABER: Recherches sur le virus de la peste aviaire pathogène pour la souris. Ses affinités pour les néoplasmes. Rev. Immunol. **3**, 5 (1937).

LEWIS, M. R., and P. M. APTEKMAN: Antigenicity of sarcomata undergoing atrophy in rats. J. Immunol. **67**, 193 (1951).

LILLY, F., E. A. BOYSE, and L. J. OLD: Genetic basis of susceptibility to viral leukaemogenesis. Lancet 1964/ii, 1207.

LINDENMANN, J.: Resistance of mice to mouse-adapted influenza A virus. Virology **16**, 203 (1962).

— Viral oncolysis with host survival. Proc. Soc. exp. Biol. (N. Y.) **113**, 85 (1963).

— Inheritance of resistance to influenza virus in mice. Proc. Soc. exp. Biol. (N. Y.) **116**, 506 (1964 a).

— Immunity to transplantable tumors following viral oncolysis. I. Mechanism of immunity to Ehrlich ascites tumor. J. Immunol, **92**, 912 (1964 b).

—, and P. A. KLEIN: Mouse tissue isoantigen detectable by immunoprecipitation. Proc. Soc. exp. Biol. (N. Y.) **117**, 446 (1964).

— — Immunity to transplantable tumors following viral oncolysis. II. Antigenic similarities between three unspecific mouse tumors. J. Immunol. **94**, 461 (1965).

— — Further studies on the resistance of mice to myxoviruses. Arch. Virusforsch. **19**, 1 (1966).

—, C. A. LANE, and D. HOBSON: The resistance of A2G mice to myxoviruses. J. Immunol. **90**, 942 (1963).

LIU, C., and F. B. BANG: Encephalitis and pneumonia following the intranasal inoculation of Newcastle disease virus in different strains of mice. Amer. J. Hyg. **55**, 182 (1952).

LUND, H. J. C.: Vaccination of rats against the Yoshida ascites sarcoma with the formation of complement-fixing antibody. Brit. J. Cancer **11**, 475 (1957).

— Vaccination of rats against the Yoshida ascites sarcoma. The antigenic relation between Yoshida's ascites sarcoma and the placenta from various species. Vaccination of rats with homologous placental tissue. Acta path. microbiol. scand. **50**, 369 (1960).

LURIA, S. E.: Viruses as determinants of cellular functions. Canad. Cancer Conf. **3**, 261 (1959).

LYNCH, C. J., and T. P. HUGHES: The inheritance of susceptibility to yellow fever encephalitis in mice. Genetics 21, 104 (1936).

MALMGREN, R. A., A. S. RABSON, and P. G. CARNEY: Immunity and viral carcinogenesis. Effect of thymectomy on polyoma virus carcinogenesis in mice. J. Nat. Cancer Inst. **33**, 101 (1964).

MANSON, L. A., G. U. FOSCHI, and J. PALM: An association of transplantation antigens with microsomal lipoproteins of normal and malignant tissues. J. cell. comp. Physiol. **61**, 109 (1963).

MARBROOK, J., and R. E. F. MATTHEWS: The differential immunogenicity of plant viral proteins and nucleoproteins. Virology **28**, 219 (1966).

McDEVITT, H. O., and M. SELA: Genetic control of the antibody response. I. Demonstration of determinant-specific differences in response to synthetic polypeptide antigens in two strains of inbred mice. J. exp. Med. **122**, 517 (1965).

McGREGOR, D. D., and J. L. GOWANS: The antibody response of rats depleted of lymphocytes by chronic drainage from the thoracic duct. J. exp. Med. **117**, 303 (1963).

McKEE, R. W., E. GARCIA, M. R. TROEH, and W. SCHULTZ: Establishment of resistance to the growth of Ehrlich ascites carcinoma in C57Black mice. Acta UICC **15**, 955 (1959).

McKENNA, J. M., R. P. SANDERSON, and W. S. BLAKEMORE: Extraction of distinctive antigens from malignant tissues. Science **135**, 370 (1962).

MEDAWAR, P. B.: The immunology of transplantation. The Harvey Lectures 1956/57, Academic Press, New York 1958.

MERRITT, K., and A. G. JOHNSON: Studies on the adjuvant action of bacterial endotoxins on antibody formation. VI. Enhancement of antibody formation by nucleic acids. J. Immunol. **94**, 416 (1965).

METZGAR, R. S.: Human pancreas-specific isoantigens. Nature (Lond.) **203**, 660 (1964).

MIKULSKA, Z. B., C. SMITH, and P. ALEXANDER: Evidence for an immunological reaction of the host directed against its own actively growing primary tumor. J. Nat. Cancer Inst. **36**, 29 (1966).

MILLER, J. F. A. P.: The thymus and the development of immunologic responsiveness. Science **144**, 1544 (1964).

MISHELL, R. I., L. A. HERZENBERG, and L. A. HERZENBERG: Leucocyte agglutination in mice. Detection of H-2 and non-H-2 isoantigens. J. Immunol. **90**, 628 (1963).

MITCHISON, N. A.: Studies on the immunological response to foreign tumor transplants in the mouse. I. The role of lymph node cells in conferring immunity by adoptive transfer. J. exp. Med. **102**, 157 (1955).

MÖLLER, E.: Isoantigenic properties of tumours transgressing histocompatibility barriers of the H-2 system. J. Nat. Cancer Inst. **33**, 979 (1964).

— Antagonistic effects of humoral isoantibodies on the in vitro cytotoxicity of immune lymphoid cells. J. exp. Med. **122**, 11 (1965 a).

— Interaction between tumor and host during progressive neoplastic growth in histoincompatible recipients. J. Nat. Cancer Inst. **35**, 1053 (1965 b).

—, and G. MÖLLER: Quantitative studies on the sensitivity of normal and neoplastic cells to the cytotoxic action of isoantibodies. J. exp. Med. **115**, 527 (1962).

MÖLLER, G.: Survival of H-2 incompatible mouse erythrocytes in untreated isoimmune recipients. Immunology **8**, 360 (1965).

—, and E. MÖLLER: Plaque-formation by non-immune and X-irradiated lymphoid cells on monolayers of mouse embryo cells. Nature (Lond.) **208**, 260 (1965).

MOLOMUT, N., M. PADNOS, V. SATORY, and L. GROSS: Survival of Ehrlich's ascites carcinoma cells at high ultra-centrifugal forces. Nature **203**, 740 (1964).

MOORE, A. E.: Destruction of sarcoma 180 by Russian encephalitis virus with host survival. Proc. Am. Ass. Cancer Res. **1**, 39 (1953).

— Effect of viruses on tumors. Ann. Rev. Microbiol. **8**, 393 (1954).

— The oncolytic viruses. Progr. exp. Tumor Res. **1**, 411 (1960).

MORGAN, C., H. M. ROSE, and D. H. MOORE: Structure and development of viruses observed in the electron microscope. III. Influenza virus. J. exp. Med. **104**, 171 (1956).

NELSON, J. B.: Response of mice to reovirus type 3 in presence and absence of ascites tumor cells. Proc. Soc. exp. Biol. (N. Y.) **116**, 1086 (1964).

—, and G. S. TARNOWSKI: An oncolytic virus recovered from Swiss mice during passage of an ascites tumour. Nature (Lond.) **188**, 866 (1960).

NELSON, R. A. Jr.: The role of complement in immune phenomena. The Inflammatory Process (ZWEIFACH, B. W., L. GRANT, and R. F. McCLUSKEY ed.) Academic Press, New York 1965.

NOSSAL, G. J. V.: The mechanism of action of antigen. Australasian Ann. Med. **14**, 321 (1965).

NOTKINS, A. L., S. E. MERGENHAGEN, A. A. RIZZO, C. SCHEELE, and T. A. WALDMANN: Elevated γ-globulin and increased antibody production in mice infected with lactic dehydrogenase virus. J. exp. Med. **123**, 347 (1966).

ODAKA, T., and T. YAMAMOTO: Inheritance of susceptibility to Friend mouse leukemia virus. Jap. J. exp. Med. **32**, 405 (1962).

— — Inheritance of susceptibility to Friend mouse leukemia virus. II. Spleen foci method applied to test the susceptibility of crossbred progeny between a sensitive and a resistant strain. Jap. J. exp. Med. **35**, 311 (1965).

OLD, L. J., and E. A. BOYSE: Immunology of experimental tumors. Ann. Rev. Med. **15**, 167 (1964).

— — Antigens of tumors and leukemias induced by viruses. Fed. Proc. **24**, 1009 (1965).

— —, and E. STOCKERT: The G (Gross) leukemia antigen. Cancer Res. **25**, 813 (1965).

PEREIRA, H. G., B. TUMOVA, and V. G. LAW: Avian influenza A viruses. Bull. Wld Hlth Org. **32**, 855 (1965).

PEREZ-TAMAYO, R., and P. R. KRETSCHMER: Inflammation in homograft rejection. The inflammatory process (ZWEIFACH, B. W., L. GRANT, and R. T. McCLUSKEY, ed.). New York: Academic Press 1965.

PERKINS, E. H., and T. MAKINODAN: The suppressive role of mouse peritoneal phagocytes in agglutinin response. J. Immunol. **94**, 765 (1965).

Petri, M.: The occurrence of Nosema cuniculi (Encephalitozoon cuniculi) in the cells of transplantable, malignant ascites tumours and its effect upon tumour and host. Acta path. microbiol. scand. **66**, 13 (1966).

Pinchuck, P., and P. H. Maurer: Antigenicity of polypeptides (poly alpha amino acids). XVI. Genetic control of immunogenicity of synthetic polypeptides in mice. J. exp. Med. **122**, 673 (1965).

Polglase, W. J.: Immunization against Ehrlich's ascites carcinoma with Streptomycin complexes from tumour cells. Nature (Lond.) **197**, 301 (1963).

Potter, J. R.: Biochemical perspectives in cancer research. Cancer Res. **24**, 1085 (1964).

Prehn, R. T.: Cancer antigens in tumors induced by chemicals. Fed. Proc. **24**, 1018 (1965).

—, and J. M. Main: Immunity to methylcholanthrene-induced sarcomas. J. Nat. Cancer Inst. **18**, 769 (1957).

Révész, L.: Effect of irradiation on the growth of the Ehrlich ascites tumor. J. Nat. Cancer Inst. **15**, 1691 (1955).

Roberts, J. A.: Growth of virulent and attenuated ectromelia virus in cultured macrophages from normal and ectromelia-immune mice. J. Immunol. **92**, 837 (1964).

Sabin, A. B.: Nature of inherited resistance to viruses affecting the nervous system. Proc. Nat. Acad. Sci. **38**, 540 (1952 a).

— Genetic factors affecting susceptibility and resistance to virus diseases of the nervous Sci. **54**, 936 (1952 b).

— Genetic factors affecting susceptibility and resistance to virus diseases of the nervous system. Proc. Ass. Res. nerv. ment. Dis. **38**, 57 (1954).

— Discussion remark. Texas Rep. Biol. Med. **15**, 599 (1957).

Sawyer, W. A., and W. Lloyd: The use of mice in tests of immunity against yellow fever. J. exp. Med. **54**, 533 (1931).

Sbarra, A. J., W. Shirley, and W. A. Bradawil: "Piggy-back" phagocytosis. Nature (Lond.) **194**, 255 (1962).

Schell, K.: Studies on the innate resistance of mice to infection with mousepox. I. Resistance and antibody production. Austr. J. exp. Biol. **38**, 271 (1960).

Schreffler, D. C.: A serologically detected variant in mouse serum: Further evidence for genetic control by the histocompatibility-2 locus. Genetics **49**, 973 (1964).

Sela, M., and E. Mozes: Dependence of the chemical nature of antibodies on the net electrical charge of antigens. Proc. Nat. Acad. Sci. **55**, 445 (1966).

Seydel, H. G.: Haemorrhage in Ehrlich ascites tumours. Nature (Lond.) **206**, 206 (1965).

Sharpless, G. R., M. C. Davies, and H. R. Cox: Antagonistic action of certain neurotropic viruses toward a lymphoid tumor in chickens with resulting immunity. Proc. Soc. exp. Biol. (N. Y.) **73**, 270 (1950).

Siegert, R.: Die onkolytischen Eigenschaften von Vieren. Arch. Virusforsch. **6**, 93 (1955).

Simpson, R. W., and G. K. Hirst: Genetic recombination among influenza viruses. I. Cross reactivation of plaque-forming capacity as a method for selecting recombinants from the progeny of crosses between influenza A strains. Virology **15**, 436 (1961).

Siskind, G. W., and H. Eisen: Effect of variation in antibody-hapten association constant upon the biologic activity of the antibody. J. Immunol. **95**, 436 (1965).

Sjögren, H. O.: Transplantation methods as a tool for detection of tumor-specific antigens. Progr. exp. Tumor Res. **6**, 289 (1965).

—, I. Hellström, and G. Klein: Transplantation of polyoma virus-induced tumors in mice. Cancer Res. **21**, 329 (1961).

Snell, G. D.: Methods for the study of histocompatibility genes. J. Genetics **49**, 87 (1948).

— Histocompatibility genes of the mouse. II. Production and analysis of isogenic resistant lines. J. Nat. Cancer Instr. **21**, 843 (1958).

— Congenic resistant strains of mice. Bar Harbor: Jackson Lab. Publication 1965.

Southam, C. M.: Present status of oncolytic virus studies. Trans. N. Y. Acad. Sci. Ser. II 22, 657 (1960).

Speir, R. W., and C. M. Southam: Interference of Newcastle disease virus with neuropathogenicity of oncolytic viruses in mice. Ann. N. Y. Acad. Sci. **83**, 551 (1960).

SPIEGELBERG, H. L., and W. O. WEIGLE: The catabolism of homologous and heterologous 7SγG fragments. J. exp. Med. 121, 323 (1965).

STAATS, J.: Standardized nomenclature for inbred strains of mice. Third listing. Cancer Res. 24, 147 (1964).

STETSON, C. A.: The role of humoral antibody in the homograft reaction. Adv. Immunol. 3, 97 (1963).

STROBER, S., and J. L. GOWANS: The role of the lymphocytes in the sensitization of rats to renal homografts. J. exp. Med. 122, 347 (1965).

STUART, A. E., and A. M. EL HASSAN: Specific inhibition of Landschütz ascites tumour by an isogenic cellular system. Lancet 1964/i, 913.

STUART-HARRIS, C. H.: A neurotropic strain of human influenza virus. Lancet 1939/i, 497.

STUCK, B., E. A. BOYSE, L. J. OLD, and E. A. CARSWELL: ML: A new antigen found in leukemias and mammary tumors of the mouse. Nature (Lond.) 203, 1033 (1964 a).

—, L. J. OLD, and E. A. BOYSE: Occurrence of soluble antigen in the plasma of mice with virus-induced leukemia. Proc. Nat. Acad. Sci. 52, 950 (1964 b).

SVET-MOLDAVSKY, G. J., and V. P. HAMBURG: Quantitative relationships in viral oncolysis and the possibility of artificial heterogenization of tumours. Nature (Lond.) 202, 303 (1964).

TEE, D. E. H., M. WANG, and J. WATKINS: Antigenic properties of human tumours. Nature (Lond.) 204, 897 (1964).

—, J. WATKINS, and M. WANG: Breakdown rate of serum 7Sγ-globulins in mice. Nature (Lond.) 208, 251 (1965).

TEMIN, H. M.: Genetic and possible biochemical mechanisms of viral carcinogenesis. Cancer Res. 26, 212 (1966).

TENNANT, J. R.: Susceptibility and resistance to viral leukemogenesis in the mouse. II. Response to the virus relative to histocompatibility factors carried by the prospective host. J. Nat. Cancer Inst. 34, 633 (1965).

TENNANT, R. W., J. C. PARKER, and T. G. WARD: Virus studies with germfree mice. II. Comparative responses of germfree mice to virus infection. J. Nat. Cancer Inst. 34, 381 (1965).

THEIS, G. A., R. E. BILLINGHAM, W. K. SILVERS, and H. KOPROWSKI: Mechanism of natural resistance of mice to virus infection. Virology 8, 264 (1959).

TRENTIN, J. J.: An outbreak of mouse-pox (infectious ectromelia) in the United States: I. Presumptive diagnosis. Science 117, 226 (1953).

—, and E. BRYAN: Immunization of hamsters and histoisogenic mice against transplantation of tumors induced by human adenovirus type 12. Proc. Amer. Ass. Cancer Res. 5, 64 (1964).

TYRRELL, D. A. J.: New tissue culture systems for influenza, Newcastle disease and vaccinia viruses. J. Immunol. 74, 293 (1955).

UHR, J. W., and G. WEISSMANN: Intracellular distribution and degradation of bacteriophage in mammalian tissues. J. Immunol. 94, 544 (1965).

UNGAR, J., and B. BASIL: Routine experience of the mouse-protection assay of pertussis vaccine. J. Hyg. (Camb.) 55, 45 (1957).

VAINIO, T., R. GWATKIN, and H. KOPROWSKI: Production of interferon by brains of genetically resistant and susceptible mice infected with West Nile virus. Virology 14, 385 (1961).

VAUGHN, R. B.: Interactions of macrophages and erythrocytes: Some further experiments. Immunology 8, 245 (1965).

VOISIN, G.-A.: Greffes tumorales et facilitation immunologique ("immunological enhancement"). Revue critique. Rev. franç. Et. Clin. Biol. 8, 927 (1963).

WAGNER, R. R.: Influenza virus infection of transplanted tumors. I. Multiplication of a "neurotropic" strain and its effect on solid neoplasms. Cancer Res. 14, 377 (1954).

— A pantropic strain of influenza virus: Generalized infection and viremia in the infant mouse. Virology 1, 497 (1955).

WEBB, H. E., G. WETHERLEY-MEIN, C. E. GORDON SMITH, and D. McMAHON: Leukaemia and neoplastic processes treated with Langat and Kyasanur forest disease viruses: A clinical and laboratory study of 28 patients. Brit. med. J. 1966/i, 258.

WEBER, W. T., P. C. NOWELL, and W. C. D. HARE: Chromosome studies on a transplanted and a primary canine venereal sarcoma. J. Nat. Cancer Inst. 35, 537 (1965).

WEBSTER, L. T.: Inheritance of resistance of mice to enteric bacterial and neurotropic virus infections. J. exp. Med. 65, 261 (1937).

—, and A. D. CLOW: Experimental encephalitis (St. Louis type) in mice with high inborn resistance. J. exp. Med. 63, 827 (1936).

—, and M. S. JOHNSON: Comparative virulence of St. Louis encephalitis virus cultured with brain tissue from innately susceptible and innately resistant mice. J. exp. Med. 74, 489 (1941).

WHEELOCK, E. F., and J. H. DINGLE: Observations on the repeated administration of viruses to a patient with acute leukemia. A preliminary report. New Engl. J. Med. 271, 645 (1964).

WHITE, R. G.: Factors affecting the antibody response. Brit. med. Bull. 19, 207 (1963).

WOGLOM, W. H.: Immunity to transplantable tumours. Cancer Rev. 4, 129 (1929).

ODARTCHENKO, N., Lausanne: Prolifération cellulaire érythropiétique.

PACK, G. T., New York: Clinical Aspects of Cancer Immunity and Cancer Susceptibility.

PACK, G. T., New York / A. H. ISLAMI, New York: Tumors of the Liver.

RITZMAN, S. E., Galveston / W. C. LEVIN, Galveston: The Syndrome of Macroglobuli-
nemia.

STEWARD, J. K., Manchester: Tumors in Children.

WEIL, R., Lausanne: Biological and Structural Properties of Polyoma Virus and its
DNA.

ZILBER, L. A., Moskva: Virogenetic Theory of Cancer Origin.